Acknowledgements

I would like to thank the following people for their significant contribution to the text: Jill Elbourn, Dr Lorraine Cale and Ken Black. Additional contributors I'd like to thank are the members of the HRE Working Group, Dr Dawn Penney, Professor Ken Fox, Professor Stuart Biddle, HMI, and all of the primary and secondary school teachers and trainee physical education teachers who contributed constructive comment.

This text was initiated within and supported by the Higher Education Institutes/ Schools Partnership Network. It is endorsed by the Physical Education Association of the UK, the British Association of Advisers and Lecturers in Physical Education, Sport England, the Youth Sport Trust and the Health Education Authority.

About the Author

Jo Harris, PhD, is a senior lecturer in physical education at Loughborough University in Leicestershire, where she has played a major role in the training of physical educators since 1990. Before that, she was involved in teacher education in Cheltenham for 2 years and taught physical education and health education at the secondary school level for 12 years. She was co-director of the Loughborough Summer School course titled 'Health-Related Exercise in the National Curriculum'. She holds a master's degree in physical education from Birmingham University and a PhD in pedagogy, exercise and children's health from Loughborough University.

Contents

Jo Harris
Loughborough University

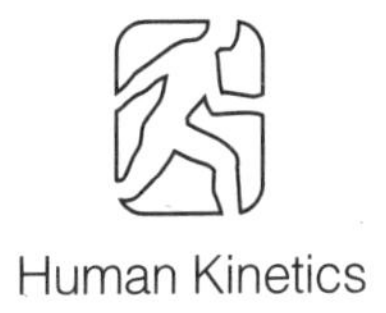

ISBN: 0-7360-0168-9

Acquisitions Editor: Scott Wikgren; **Developmental Editor:** Katy M. Patterson; **Assistant Editor:** Amanda S. Ewing; **Copyeditor:** Bob Replinger; **Proofreader:** Erin T. Cler; **Graphic Designer:** Fred Starbird; **Graphic Artist:** Kathleen Boudreau-Fuoss; **Photo Manager:** Clark Brooks; **Cover Designer:** Jack W. Davis; **Photographer (interior):** Remi Gauvain and Jo Harris; **Printer:** Creative Print and Design Group

Printed in the United Kingdom 10 9 8 7 6 5 4 3 2

Human Kinetics
Web site: www.humankinetics.com

United States: Human Kinetics, P.O. Box 5076, Champaign, IL 61825-5076
800-747-4457
e-mail: humank@hkusa.com

Canada: Human Kinetics, 475 Devonshire Road, Unit 100, Windsor, ON N8Y 2L5
800-465-7301 (in Canada only)
e-mail: orders@hkcanada.com

Europe: Human Kinetics, 107 Bradford Road, Stanningley
Leeds LS28 6AT, United Kingdom
+44 (0) 113 255 5665
e-mail: hk@hkeurope.com

Australia: Human Kinetics, 57A Price Avenue, Lower Mitcham, South Australia 5062
08 8277 1555
e-mail: liahka@senet.com.au

New Zealand: Human Kinetics, P.O. Box 105-231, Auckland Central
09-523-3462
e-mail: hkp@ihug.co.nz

Health-Related Exercise Working Group

Chair

Jo Harris
Loughborough University
Physical Education Association
of the United Kingdom

Members (in alphabetical order)

Len Almond
Loughborough University; past director of the HEA Health and Physical Education Project (1985–1992)

Keith Bailey
Roding Valley High School, Essex

Barry Benn
Westhill College, Birmingham

Sean Bettinson
Emanuel School, London

Ken Black
Disability sport officer, Youth Sport Trust

Elaine Burgess
Sport England

Lorraine Cale
Loughborough University

Sue Chedzoy
Exeter University

Rachel Cook
Burleigh Community College, Leicestershire

Jill Edwards
Turves Green Junior and Infant School, Birmingham

Jill Elbourn
Educational Exercise Consultant; formerly an executive member of the Physical Education Association of the United Kingdom

David Geldart
Saint Mary's Catholic Comprehensive School (Sports College), Leeds, West Yorkshire

Kevin Gilliver
Physical Education Association of the United Kingdom; formerly PE officer at Qualifications, Curriculum and Assessment Authority (QCA)

Michael Gray
Leeds Metropolitan University

Maura Hyland
St. Peters High School and Sixth Form Centre, Gloucester

Peter Lamb
Raincliffe School, Scarborough

Bob Laventure
Physical activity and health promotion consultant (formerly with the Health Education Authority)

Alan Lindsay
BAALPE; PE advisory teacher, Suffolk

Stewart McKenzie
PE adviser, West Sussex; formerly University of Brighton (Chelsea School)

Stephen Pain
Inspector for PE and SEN, Wandsworth, London

Helen Queen
De Montfort University

Stephen Pain
Inspector for PE and SEN,
Wandsworth, London

Helen Queen
De Montfort University

Lynne Spackman
Awdurdod Cymwysterau
Cwricwlwm Ac Asesu Cymru
(Qualifications, Curriculum and
Assessment Authority for Wales)
(ACCAC)

Gareth Stratton
Liverpool John Moores University

Mike Waring
University of Durham

Angela Wortley
University of Leicester

Martin Yelling
De Montfort University

Introduction

HOW CAN THIS GUIDANCE MATERIAL BE USED?

This guidance material focuses specifically on health issues within physical education (PE) although appropriate links are made with relevant health-related aspects of personal, social and health education (PSHE) and science. The guidance material focuses on physical activity as a desirable health-related behaviour and assists teachers in planning, delivering and evaluating a structured, coherent and comprehensive health-related exercise programme that helps young people value and benefit from an active lifestyle.

The guidance material is presented in the following six sections: terminology, rationale and recommendations, delivery and assessment, requirements and approaches, example scheme and units of work, and resources and contacts.

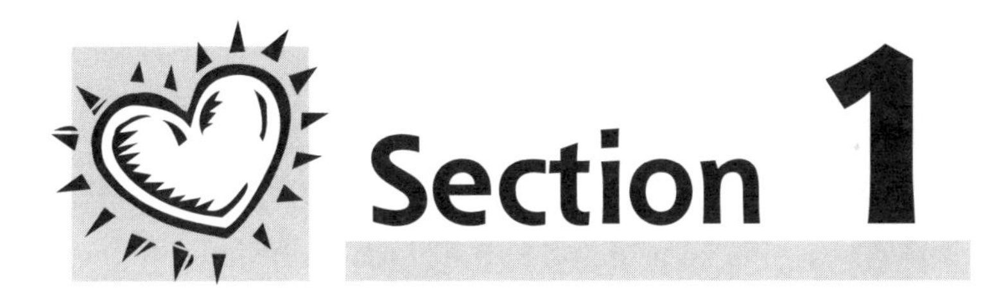

Section 1

Terminology

WHAT IS HEALTH, HEALTH PROMOTION AND HEALTH EDUCATION?

Health is a positive state of physical, mental and social well-being.

Health promotion involves disease prevention, risk reduction and the optimisation of health.

Health education is any activity designed to achieve health-related learning. Effective health education can produce changes in knowledge and understanding, influence values and attitudes, facilitate the acquisition of skills and affect lifestyle changes.

WHAT IS PHYSICAL ACTIVITY, EXERCISE AND FITNESS?

Physical activity is any bodily movement produced by muscles that results in energy expenditure. This includes all forms of active play, sport, dance and exercise as well as active transportation (walking, cycling) and routine habitual activities (housework, gardening).

Exercise is planned, structured physical activity that enhances aspects of physical, mental and social health and fitness and well-being.

Fitness is a capacity or a set of attributes that individuals have or achieve that enable them to participate in and benefit from physical activity. Fitness has physical and mental dimensions.

Fitness for life, fitness for health and **health-related fitness** all refer to the physical and mental dimensions of fitness that are considered to have implications for health, examples of the latter being reduced risk of coronary heart disease, back pain, osteoporosis, obesity, depression and anxiety. These dimensions include cardiovascular efficiency, muscular strength and endurance, flexibility, body composition, composure and decision-making.

Fitness for performance and **skill-related fitness** both refer to the physical and mental dimensions of fitness that are considered to have implications for sport performance. These dimensions include agility, balance, co-ordination, power, reaction time, speed, concentration and determination.

WHAT IS HEALTH-RELATED EXERCISE?

Health-related exercise (HRE) is physical activity associated with health enhancement. Within the context of the National Curriculum for Physical Education, HRE relates to the contribution of physical education to health and its expression within the curriculum. Delivery of this area includes the teaching of knowledge, understanding, physical competence and behavioural skills, and the creation of positive attitudes and confidence associated with current and lifelong participation in physical activity. Within the subject of physical education, the most appropriate teaching approaches involve learning through *active* participation in purposeful physical activity embracing a range of sport, dance and exercise experiences including individualised lifetime activities.

WHY ARE THERE DIFFERENT HEALTH-RELATED TERMS?

Numerous terms have been used for the area associated with the contribution of physical education to health, examples being health-related fitness (HRF), health-related physical fitness (HRPF), health-related physical education (HRPE), health-based physical education (HBPE), health-focused physical education (HFPE) and a health focus in physical education. These different terms reflect the varying influences on health issues within physical education over time. Within this text, health-related exercise (HRE) has been adopted as the most appropriate term for health issues associated with physical activity within the school curriculum.

Within public health arenas, a shift has occurred towards use of the terms health-related physical activity (HRPA) and health-enhancing physical activity (HEPA) to highlight the wide range of moderate-intensity routine physical activities such as walking, gardening and housework (besides more structured forms of exercise and sport) that contribute to health.

WHAT IS THE RELATIONSHIP AMONG PHYSICAL ACTIVITY, FITNESS AND HEALTH?

Over the years there has been a shift in emphasis from hard training to improve fitness scores towards enjoyable participation in physical activity for health benefits. The current focus is on the process of being active, not solely reaching a state of fitness. One of the reasons for this shift has been the recognition that exercise does not have to be strenuous to produce health benefits and does not have to hurt to provide benefits. Research indicates that moderate levels of physical activity (equivalent in intensity to brisk walking) have beneficial effects on an individual's health (for example, improved mental health and reduced risk of heart disease), and such benefits may occur as a consequence of physical activity levels that are well below the intensity necessary for fitness changes. Indeed, research suggests that the total amount of physical activity (measured in energy expenditure) is the important factor when considering health benefits (rather than simply the intensity of the activity).

The key public health message is that it is not essential to undertake high-intensity exercise to achieve health benefits. Associated public health messages include the following:

No pain and you still gain.

It doesn't have to be hell to be healthy.

Some exercise is better than none.

Furthermore, regular physical activity is related to physical, mental and social health benefits, independent of fitness levels. For children, the link between activity levels and health appears stronger than that between fitness and health. Every child can benefit from being active but not every child can reach a high level of fitness because the latter is constrained by genetic limitations, maturational status and trainability. Indeed, even if they train at a high level over a period, some children may achieve only insignificant improvement of their fitness levels.

In addition, if a child can increase fitness, she can only achieve it by becoming more active. Many children will never be able to run a mile in 6 minutes or perform 10 pull-ups even if they train hard and do their best. They can, however, increase the number of times that they walk, jog or cycle at a comfortable pace and the length of time they do this. Most important, being active for 30 to 60 minutes every day is a desirable and attainable target for every child (figure 1.1). It is also known that physically active children are more likely to become physically active adults.

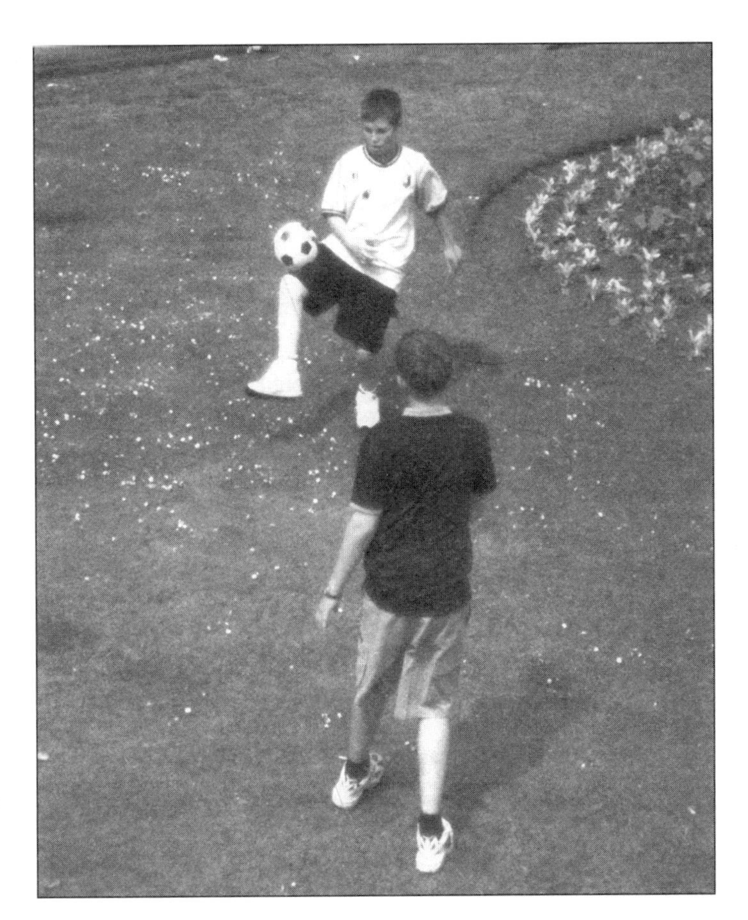

Figure 1.1 Football is one of many activities that pupils can participate in that helps them to be active for 30-60 minutes each day.

In summary, from a health perspective, increasing activity levels will bring associated health benefits and may enhance fitness.

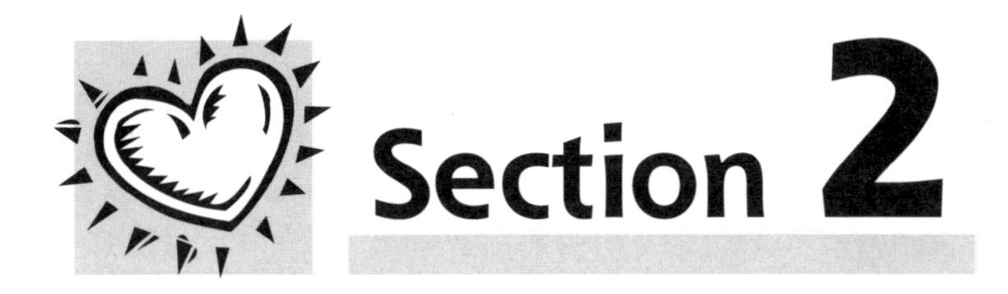

Section 2

Rationale and Recommendations

WHY SHOULD SCHOOLS PROMOTE PHYSICAL ACTIVITY?

Schools should promote physical activity for the following reasons:

- » Physical activity has a beneficial effect on the physical, mental and social health of young people.
- » Some young people have risk factors for chronic conditions such as heart disease, and obesity is becoming more prevalent among children and adolescents.
- » People often acquire and establish patterns of health-related behaviours during childhood and adolescence.
- » Many children are relatively inactive (with girls being less active than boys at all ages).
- » Physical activity declines during adolescence (this being especially dramatic with girls).
- » Schools are an efficient vehicle for providing physical activity programmes because they reach virtually all children and adolescents.
- » Schools have the potential to improve the health of young people by providing programmes and services that promote enjoyable, lifelong physical activity.
- » School programmes have successfully promoted young people's knowledge and understanding of physical activity, their attitudes towards physical education and physical activity, and their activity and fitness levels.

How Can Schools Promote Physical Activity?

To promote physical activity, it is recommended that schools

- » establish a whole-school approach to the promotion of enjoyable, lifelong physical activity among young people;
- » provide physical and social environments that encourage and enable safe, enjoyable physical activity;
- » make a commitment to health-related exercise within the national curriculum by implementing structured and co-ordinated programmes of study that

emphasise enjoyable participation in physical activity and help pupils develop the knowledge, understanding, physical competence, behavioural skills, positive attitudes and confidence needed to adopt and maintain physically active lifestyles;

- provide curricular (entitlement) and extra-curricular (extension and enrichment) physical activity programmes that meet the needs and interests of all pupils, including those who are the least active, those who are physically less competent and those with special educational needs;
- contribute to the provision of support and training for individuals involved in imparting the knowledge, skills and attitudes needed to promote enjoyable, lifelong physical activity among young people; and
- collaborate with families and community organisations to develop, implement and evaluate physical activity programmes for young people.

What Is a Whole-School Approach to Promoting Physical Activity?

Although the curriculum is a vitally important vehicle for delivering health education, it is only one avenue for the promotion of a healthy, active lifestyle. Many aspects of a school can either promote or inhibit health-related behaviours, and the understanding gained through the curriculum can either be reinforced and supported or completely undermined. The promotion of healthy patterns of behaviour requires health education to permeate the ethos of a school as well as to be a part of the formal curriculum. Health education in schools does not begin and end in the classroom; the subtle messages pupils receive about health from the daily life of school are as important as those given during lessons. Consequently, a whole-school approach to the promotion of a healthy, active lifestyle is recommended to ensure coherence and consistency for pupils. This entails exploring the potential of every aspect of the school environment to promote a healthy, active lifestyle. Examples of whole-school initiatives include the Healthy School and the Active School.

A **Healthy School** aims to achieve healthy lifestyles for the entire school population (pupils, staff, governors and parents) by developing supportive environments conducive to the promotion of health. A Healthy School is expected to make explicit its commitment to health by highlighting aspects of learning that promote good health through its curricular, extracurricular and organisational practices. A Healthy School is one that is successful in helping pupils do their best and build on their achievements.

An **Active School** makes a commitment to physical activity by aiming to increase the physical activity levels of the entire school population (pupils, staff, governors and parents) in a way that is likely to have a positive and sustained impact on physical activity habits even outside the physical education class (figure 2.1).

Healthy and Active Schools are expected to achieve harmonious interpersonal relationships and healthy alliances within the school and in the community.

WHAT ARE SOME EXAMPLES OF SCHOOL POLICIES?

Examples of a Healthy School policy and an Active School policy are provided on pages 7-9. Of course, individual school policies will vary and may include additional or differing aims depending on needs, resources and expertise. Teachers are encouraged to develop policies that are feasible and appropriate for their particular schools. In general, three main elements are important in policy development: the curriculum (formal and informal), the school environment (hidden curriculum) and the community.

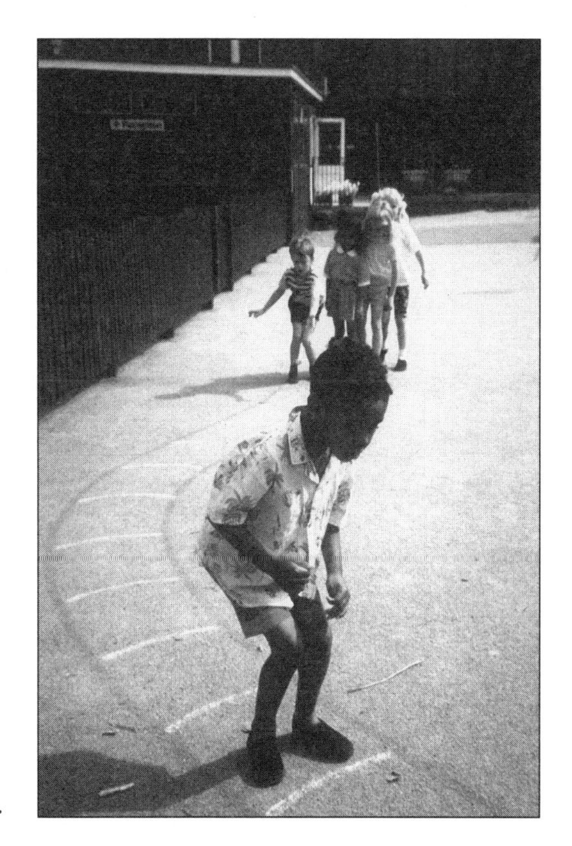

Figure 2.1 An Active School encourages physical activity not only during PE but outside of class as well.

It is possible for a school to adopt either or both of these policies or to choose to combine elements of each. Guidance on the National Healthy School Standard is available from the publications section of the Department for Education and Employment (address on page 80). More information about Active School initiatives (such as Activemark and Activemark Gold for primary schools and Sportsmark and Sportsmark Gold for secondary schools) is available from the British Heart Foundation and Sport England (addresses on pages 80 and 81).

Example: Healthy School Policy

The aim of a Healthy School policy is to achieve healthy lifestyles for the entire school population by developing an environment conducive to the promotion of health.

Curriculum—Formal and Informal

A Healthy School will

- provide a comprehensive, coherent and co-ordinated health education programme that complies with statutory requirements and is accessible to and meets the needs of all pupils;
- provide a health education programme that is well resourced and adequately staffed;
- ensure that teaching is informed and is based on a positive approach;
- monitor pupils' health-related attitudes and behaviours;
- provide an extra-curricular programme that includes a range of health-promoting lifestyle activities (e.g., physical activities, self-defence, time management, relaxation); and
- organise health-promoting events in both curricular and extra-curricular time (e.g., health days or weeks).

School Environment—Hidden Curriculum

A Healthy School will

- create a school climate in which good relationships, respect and consideration for others flourish;
- provide a clean, tidy, safe, secure and stimulating school environment;
- provide adequate toilet, cloakroom and changing facilities;
- provide a smoke-free environment;
- provide and promote healthy food choices for pupils and staff (e.g., encourage healthy packed lunches through the school caterers and tuck shops); and
- provide and promote opportunities for pupils and staff to be physically active.

Community

A Healthy School will

- raise awareness and enlist the support of staff, parents and governors to the health messages being promoted within school;
- establish and maintain links with appropriate services (e.g., health education, health promotion) and other agencies (e.g., social services, traffic safety) to advise, support and contribute to the promotion of health;
- develop partnerships with other schools, pupils, parents and the wider community on a range of health-promoting initiatives;
- provide a range of health-promoting lifestyle activities for staff, governors and parents (e.g., physical activities, self-defence, time and stress management, relaxation);
- provide pupils, staff, governors and parents with information on health matters (e.g., posters, leaflets);
- provide knowledge, understanding and opportunities for adults who work in and regularly visit school; and
- have an active policy-making committee (with pupil, staff, governor and parent representation) to develop, implement and evaluate the effectiveness of the Healthy School policy.

Example: Active School Policy

The aim of an Active School policy is to increase the activity levels of the whole school population by developing a supportive environment conducive to the promotion of physical activity.

Curriculum—Formal and Informal

An Active School will

- provide a broad, balanced and relevant physical education programme that complies with statutory requirements and is accessible to and meets the needs of all pupils;
- fully implement in practice national curriculum requirements for health-related exercise through an effectively planned, delivered and evaluated programme of study;
- provide pupils with a minimum of two hours of physical education each week of the school year;
- provide a physical education programme that is well resourced and adequately staffed;

- » monitor pupils' level of involvement in sport and activity (in and out of school);
- » provide an extra-curricular programme that includes a range of purposeful and enjoyable physical activities (competitive and non-competitive, team and individual, recreational);
- » increase the proportion of pupils who regularly participate in extra-curricular activities;
- » increase the proportion of staff who regularly contribute to the extra-curricular programme; and
- » organise events (both in curricular and extra-curricular time) that promote physical activity (e.g., sports day, activity weeks, outdoor education experiences).

School Environment—Hidden Curriculum

An Active School will

- » provide safe, adequate and stimulating play areas and promote activity in these areas;
- » make sports facilities and equipment available for recreational use at lunchtimes and breaktimes;
- » increase the proportion of pupils and staff who walk or cycle to school;
- » provide secure storage areas for bicycles;
- » increase the proportion of staff who regularly participate in physical activity; and
- » provide adequate changing and showering facilities for pupils and staff.

Community

An Active School will

- » raise awareness and enlist the support of staff, parents and governors to the physical activity messages being promoted within school;
- » provide all pupils with up-to-date, accurate information about activity opportunities in their local community;
- » develop alliances and partnerships with local providers (e.g., sports clubs, leisure centres, health and fitness clubs) to increase the activity opportunities for pupils;
- » provide and lobby for opportunities for pupils, staff, governors and parents to be active (e.g., safe walking and cycling routes);
- » provide advice, guidance and counselling to pupils, staff, parents and governors who wish to become more active;
- » provide opportunities for staff and parents to gain appropriate qualifications that will enable them to become involved in and contribute to the extra-curricular programme; and
- » have an active policy-making committee (with pupil, staff, governor and parent representation) to develop, implement and evaluate the effectiveness of the Active School policy.

WHAT IS THE CONTRIBUTION OF PHYSICAL EDUCATION TO HEALTH?

Physical education makes a significant contribution to health through its focus on safe participation in health-enhancing exercise and the promotion of an active way of life. A well-structured and co-ordinated physical education programme should provide

- » a knowledge base about exercise including an understanding of (a) the effects, benefits and risks of being active, (b) safe, effective and developmentally appropriate exercise practices and (c) the opportunities and constraints associated with being active;
- » practically applied understanding of exercise in order to enhance (a) current and future health, fitness and well-being and (b) performance in sport, dance and exercise activities;
- » the opportunity to experience of a range of physical activities, including those that can be pursued throughout life (e.g., walking, jogging, swimming, aerobics, dancing);
- » behavioural skills associated with activity promotion (e.g., knowing how to go about being more active, ways of overcoming constraints to being active, strategies for maintaining involvement in physical activity);
- » enhanced attitudes, self-esteem and self-confidence in a physical activity environment; and
- » a sense of empowerment to change school and community policies and practices related to physical activity.

Health-related exercise makes an important contribution to physical education in terms of activity and health promotion and performance enhancement. HRE involves the promotion of all forms of physical activity that are safe, beneficial and enjoyable. It is a myth that HRE is anti-games, anti-sport or anti-performance. Movement ability or physical competence plus confidence is required for enjoyable and sustained participation in physical activity (figure 2.2).

Health-related exercise is a key component of physical education—it is central to and underpins the subject of physical education and serves to co-ordinate the range of experiences in physical education.

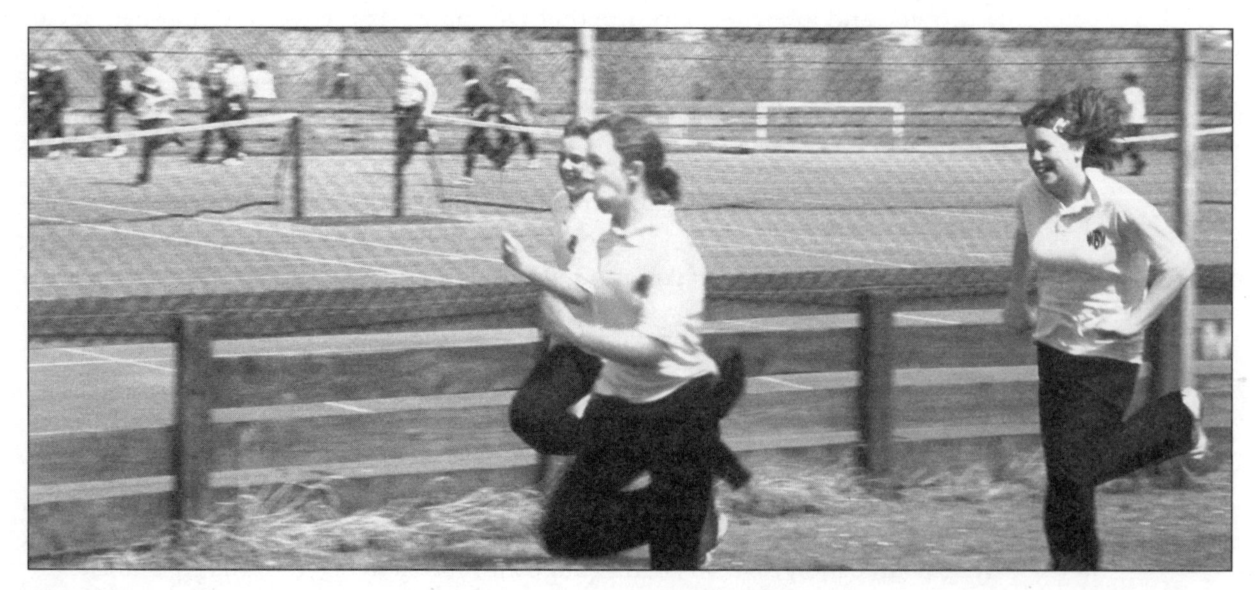

Figure 2.2 Ability and confidence are needed for an activity to be enjoyable.

WHAT IS A 'PHYSICALLY EDUCATED' YOUNG PERSON?

In terms of health-related outcomes, a 'physically educated' young person is one who:

- Has learned the skills necessary to perform a variety of physical activities:
  - Demonstrates competence in many different forms of physical activity
  - Has learned how to develop new skills
- Participates regularly in physical activity:
  - Participates in physical activity most days of the week
  - Knows how to monitor involvement in physical activity
  - Is able to plan, perform and evaluate safe personal exercise programmes
  - Knows the amount of physical activity recommended for health benefits
- Understands the implications of being involved in physical activity:
  - Identifies the benefits, costs and obligations associated with regular participation in physical activity
  - Understands safety factors associated with participation in physical activity
  - Recognises constraints to exercise and is able to develop strategies to help overcome them
  - Understands that physical activity provides opportunities for enjoyment, self-expression and communication
  - Understands that well-being involves more than just being physically active (i.e., it involves other health behaviours such as eating a balanced diet and not smoking)
- Values physical activity and its contribution to a healthy lifestyle:
  - Adopts an active way of life that helps to make the most of her abilities
  - Appreciates the relationships with others that can result from participation in physical activity
  - Cherishes the feelings that result from regular participation in physical activity
  - Understands the role that regular physical activity plays in the pursuit of lifelong health and well-being
  - Is aware and empowered to change the community and physical activity environment

WHAT DOES THIS MEAN FOR PHYSICAL EDUCATION?

To develop physically educated young people, the physical education programme must

- develop in young people a desire to be active,
- help young people to understand the importance of an active way of life,
- encourage young people to be independently active,
- assist young people in becoming informed consumers of health and fitness goods and services (e.g., video tapes, exercise equipment, testing devices),
- promote involvement in a range of physical activities, including those that appeal to young people (e.g., roller-blading, skate-boarding, dancing) and those that they can pursue throughout life such as walking, jogging, swimming, circuits and aerobics.

HOW MUCH EXERCISE SHOULD YOUNG PEOPLE DO?

To promote physical activity, teachers need to know and inform young people about how much physical activity they should be doing. The Health Development Agency (formerly the Health Education Authority) in England has developed the physical activity recommendations for young people shown in box 2.1.

Box 2.1

Physical Activity Recommendations for Young People

Major	Subsidiary
All young people should participate in physical activity of at least moderate intensity (moderate intensity exercise is equivalent to brisk walking) for one hour per day (i.e., 60 minutes accumulated during a day). Young people who currently do little activity should participate in physical activity of at least moderate intensity for at least half an hour per day (i.e., 30 minutes accumulated during a day).	At least twice a week, young people should participate in activities that help to enhance and maintain muscular strength and flexibility and bone health.

Why Has the Major Recommendation Been Developed?

The major recommendation is based on the following findings, which suggest that an increase in participation in physical activity is needed because

- childhood obesity is increasing,
- many young people possess at least one modifiable risk factor for coronary heart disease,
- many young people have symptoms of psychological distress, and
- the majority of young people are currently participating in 30 minutes of moderate physical activity per day on most days of the week.

Why Has the Subsidiary Recommendation Been Developed?

The subsidiary recommendation is based on the finding that participation in strength and weight-bearing activities increases bone mineral density and is believed to be related to reduced long-term risk of osteoporosis (a condition associated with fragile bones). Muscular strength and flexibility are considered to be particularly important because they affect the ability to perform routine activities such as lifting, carrying, pulling, pushing, reaching, bending and twisting. In particular, the strength of the back and abdominal muscles (the 'trunk' region) is considered to be associated with reduced risk of back pain and injury.

How Should These Recommendations Be Used With Young People?

The recommendations represent a shift from the traditional adult recommendation of '3 × 20 minutes vigorous exercise', which is now recognised as unnecessarily high for health benefits and inappropriate for young people. Younger children tend to have sporadic rather than sustained physical activity patterns, and they have exercise responses that differ from those of adults.

The physical activity recommendations for young people are important and helpful. Increasing young people's awareness of activity recommendations, benefits and opportunities should help them to increase their activity levels. Any increase, even small amounts, represents significant progress in public health. The recommendations should be viewed as guidelines rather than rigid prescriptions. The recommended levels should be gradually progressed over time with the starting point being the young person's current level of physical activity.

To nurture long-term participation, it is more prudent to motivate, inspire and help young people to be active (through encouragement, support and role-modelling) than to force them into activity sessions that may be uncomfortable and unpleasant. A hard-line, 'boot camp' approach is likely to be counterproductive in the long term. Short-term fitness gains should never take precedence over long-term positive changes in activity behaviour.

Is There Any Additional Guidance?

Recommendations have been made in the past relating to the amount and type of strength and stretching exercises that children should be doing. Strength and flexibility exercises are recommended for young people because they provide benefits in the form of improved posture, protection against future back pain and osteoporosis (a condition associated with fragile bones), prevention against injury and enhanced performance (figure 2.3).

Although it is possible for girls and boys (both before and after puberty) to achieve strength and flexibility gains from specific exercises (beyond what would have occurred because of natural growth and development), it is recognised that risks are associated with some forms of flexibility training and weight-training. These risks are mainly associated with poor technique, unsupervised lifting of heavy weights and extreme stretch positions, all of which cause unnecessary pain and damage. It is important that pupils understand both the benefits and the hazards associated with such forms of exercise and know how to minimise risk, prevent injury and promote good health.

To maximise the benefits and minimise the risks involved, the recommendations in box 2.2 are made with respect to strength and flexibility exercises for young people in school settings.

a

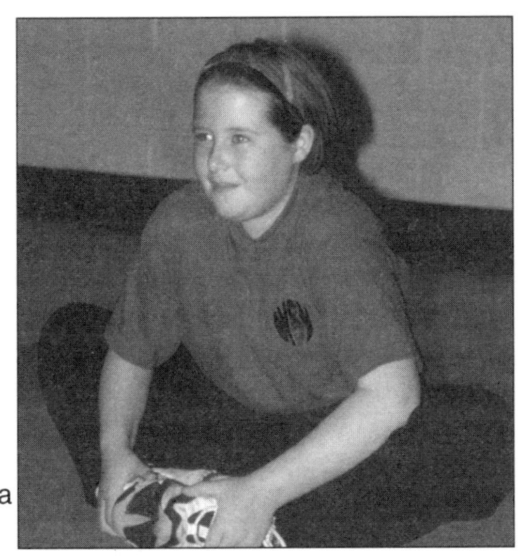

b

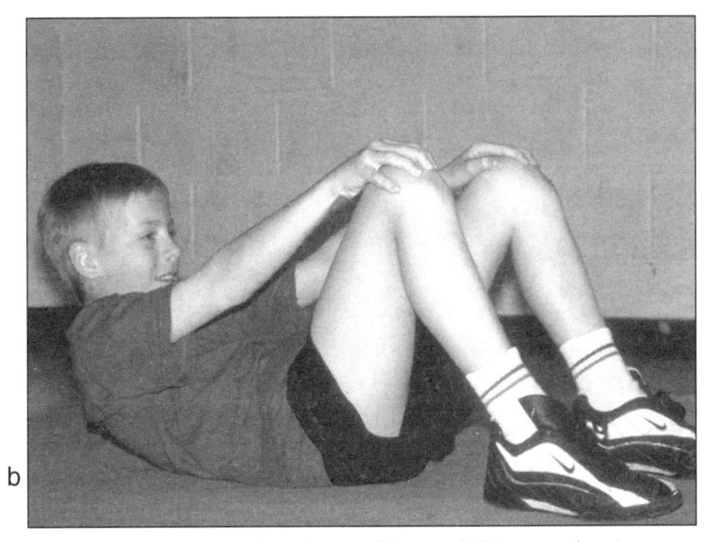

Figure 2.3 Pupils can improve their performance and help prevent injury by *(a)* stretching and *(b)* strengthening major muscle groups.

Box 2.2

Recommendations for Strength and Flexibility Exercises for Young People in School Settings

Weight or load-bearing activities are recommended for children of all ages. These include activities in which the body must support

i. all or part of its own weight (e.g., running, jumping, dancing, gymnastics), or

ii. the weight of additional objects (e.g., a throwing or striking implement such as a bat, ball, bean bag, quoit, hoop).

Primary school children should be involved in a wide range of weight-bearing activities for both the upper body (e.g., climbing, throwing, catching, striking) and the lower body (e.g., running, jumping, hopping, skipping). Older primary school children (age 9 to 11 years) can additionally be involved in developmentally appropriate low-level exercises involving their own body weight such as easy curl-ups (with legs bent and hands along floor) for the abdominal (tummy) muscles and easy push-ups (against a wall or in a box position) for muscles in the arms and chest.

Education about back care is important for both primary and secondary school children. Safe lifting, carrying and lowering involves

- getting close to the object being lifted,
- keeping a wide, solid base with feet apart and firmly on the ground,
- using the large leg muscles rather than the back muscles,
- tightening the abdominal muscles,
- keeping the back straight when lifting or lowering,
- holding the object close to the body, and
- getting assistance if the object is very heavy.

Secondary school children should be involved in differentiated exercises involving their body weight, particularly for muscles that assist good posture (i.e., the back and abdominal muscles). It is recommended that secondary school children learn how to perform body-resistance exercises with good technique before progressing to exercises involving external weights.

Secondary school children can safely use low-resistance external weights (such as light dumb-bells, elastics and tubing). Medium- to high-resistance external weights (possible with fixed equipment such as a multi-gym and with free weights such as dumb-bells and barbells) are advisable only with older secondary school children (age 14 to 18 years). Lifting near-maximal weights is appropriate only for young people age 16 to 18 years who have reached the final stage of maturation.

Young people should perform a strength exercise no more than 10 times before resting the muscles involved. They should perform unfamiliar exercises only 4 to 6 times, progressing over time to 10 repeats. Controlled lifting and lowering should be emphasised. Pupils should progress gradually from one to three sets. Each session should include exercises for a balanced range of major muscle groups. No more than three sessions a week of strength exercises are recommended, and at least one day of rest should occur between sessions. Any increase in frequency, intensity or duration should be gradual (by only 5 to 10 percent at a time).

Stretching exercises are recommended for all age groups, especially secondary school pupils. Young people should only perform stretching following cardiovascular activity when the muscles are warm. They should move into each stretch slowly and hold still. The holding time for stretches should vary from 6 to 20 seconds (depending on the weather, the warmth of the muscles, and the age and maturity of the children). Primary school children can learn simple and frequently used stretches (e.g., whole-body stretches, calf stretches), and secondary school children can learn stretches for specific muscle groups (e.g., triceps, hamstrings). It is recommended that stretches be taught within warm-ups and cool-downs. The knowledge, understanding and skills associated with stretching should be progressively taught over time.

With reference to both strength and stretching exercises, the emphasis with all age groups should be on safety and quality, not quantity, with particular attention paid to progression and balance. Young people should understand the purpose of exercises and be able to perform them with good technique and at a developmentally appropriate level (i.e., one that matches their stage of physical and psychological maturity). They should know how to make exercises easier or harder.

The learning environment should be positive and non-threatening, and the focus should be on personal improvement, not comparison with other pupils. The delivery should aim to involve young people in their own learning and promote a responsible attitude towards safe, health-enhancing exercise behaviour.

Properly designed strength and flexibility training programmes for young people should be

i. child centred and individualised, including developmentally appropriate exercises that match the physical and psychological maturity of the young person,

ii. progressive with only gradual increases in frequency, intensity or duration being made at any one time,

iii. balanced (i.e., only one part of a total exercise programme, incorporating all the major muscle groups), and

iv. competently taught and closely supervised by an appropriately qualified adult.

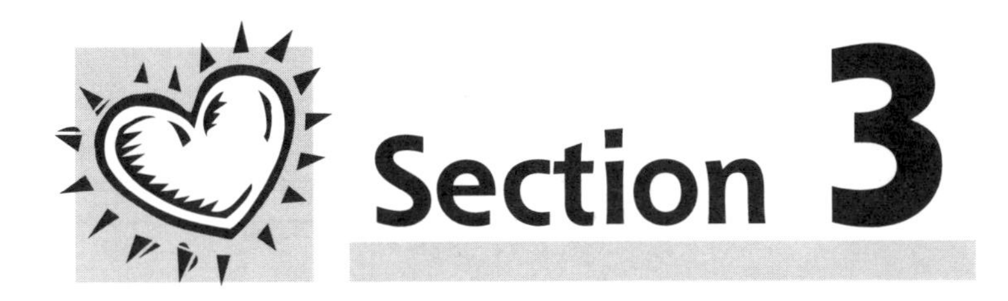

Delivery and Assessment

HOW SHOULD HRE BE DELIVERED?

To date, interpretations of HRE and its form of delivery have varied. Research has highlighted examples of narrow interpretations that equate HRE solely with vigorous activity, warming up or fitness testing. Narrow interpretations have the potential to lead to undesirable practices such as 'forced' fitness regimes, directed activity with minimal learning, inactive PE lessons involving excessive teacher talk, arduous testing, or dull, uninspiring drills.

In the past, the content of HRE courses has been dominated by physiological issues (such as the physical effects of exercise and fitness testing). There has been much less attention to psycho-social and environmental issues (such as considering the reasons why people are not active and helping individuals to overcome some of the constraints).

HRE comprises

» knowledge and understanding (cognitive domain),
» competence and motor skills (psychomotor domain),
» behavioural skills (behavioural domain), and
» attitudes and confidence (affective domain).

Given that HRE is an holistic and wide-ranging concept, its delivery demands a comprehensive range of teaching strategies and styles. Good practice requires HRE to be planned, effectively delivered and evaluated. In contrast, poor practice is unstructured, piecemeal and sporadic. Box 3.1 presents desirable and undesirable practices in the delivery of HRE.

Box 3.1

Desirable and Undesirable Practices for Delivering HRE

HRE	Desirable practices	Undesirable practices
Status	Explicit, valued, planned, evaluated	Implicit, low status, incidental, not monitored

(continued)

Box 3.1 *(continued)*

HRE	Desirable practices	Undesirable practices
Breadth and relevance	Comprehensive, meaningful; focus on health, activity, participation	Narrow, superficial; sole emphasis on fitness testing, hard training, elite performance
Coherence and status	Coherent, co-ordinated; clear links with the physical education activity areas, PSHE and related subjects; integrated	Ad hoc, hit and miss; limited links with physical education activity areas, PSHE and related subjects; isolated
Equity	Inclusive; involving all pupils	Exclusive; reduced or minimal involvement of pupils such as the least active, less competent and those with disabilities and health conditions
Action	Requires guidance and support	Requires change

Educating children about exercise and promoting lifelong participation cannot be left to chance. Children do not automatically develop the knowledge, understanding, skills, behaviours, attitudes and confidence that lead to regular participation in physical activity. These need to be taught, and this teaching must be planned.

WHAT GUIDING PRINCIPLES UNDERPIN THE TEACHING OF HRE?

The teaching of HRE involves more than just passing on information to young people. Knowing the benefits of physical activity is not sufficient to affect behaviour change. Many young people and adults know that exercise is 'good' for them, but they do not do enough exercise to gain health benefits. They need to be motivated to be active, and they need to be helped to feel good about being active. The way health-related information and experiences are taught to young people is critical. The delivery of HRE is no less important than the content.

For young people to learn to love being active and acquire a commitment to an active way of live, the delivery should embrace the following guiding principles:

- Exercise can be a positive and enjoyable experience.
- Exercise is for all.
- Everyone can benefit from exercise.
- Everyone can be good at exercise.
- Everyone can find the right kind of exercise for them.
- Exercise is for life.
- Excellence in health-related exercise is maintaining an active way of life.

Pupils should gain pleasure, enjoyment and satisfaction from their involvement in physical activity. This requires that each of them have opportunities to make progress, succeed and feel confident about being active. They should also be encouraged to help others develop a positive active image of themselves.

Young people should be helped to shift from dependence on the teacher as the activity leader to a situation in which they have acquired the understanding, competence and confidence to be independently active. They should be encouraged towards greater ownership of their activity experiences. Young people should be helped to reflect critically on their choices and actions and to develop increasing responsibility for their physical activity (figure 3.1).

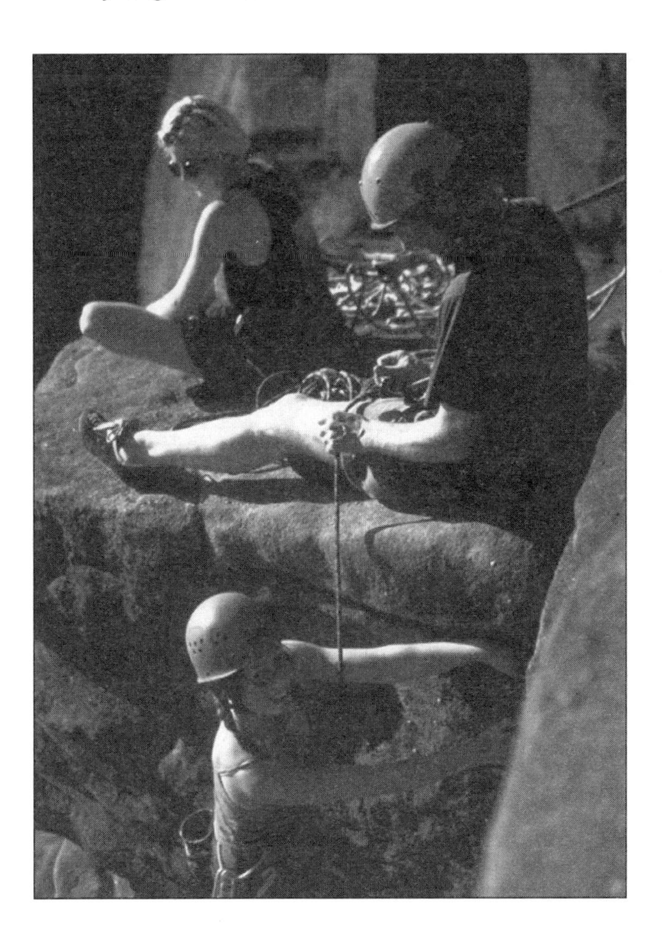

Figure 3.1 Rock climbing is an example of an individual activity that encourages and requires responsibility.

Positive experiences of physical activity are critical to the promotion of active lifestyles. Research informs us, however, that many young people are not active enough on their own time and do not have sufficient PE time in school. In addition, studies indicate that in some PE lessons children are actively moving for only about a third of the lesson. The rest of the time they are being transported to the venue, changing, listening to the teacher, queueing for equipment, waiting for their turn or are off-task. Clearly, it is desirable that pupils are more physically active during PE lessons. This can generally be addressed through improved planning and more efficient organisation and management of equipment, resources and pupils. The recommendations found in box 3.2 concern activity levels in physical education lessons.

WHAT IS 'DEVELOPMENTALLY APPROPRIATE' AND 'DIFFERENTIATED' PHYSICAL ACTIVITY?

Young people are different shapes and sizes, and pupils of the same chronological age can be as much as three to four years apart in maturation and development. In physical education, it is important to use developmentally appropriate practices that recognise children's differing and changing capacity for physical activity. A

Box 3.2

Active Physical Education Lessons

During physical education lessons, pupils should be physically active for *at least 50 percent* of the available lesson time. The activity should be purposeful and the experience positive.

When not physically active, pupils should be involved in tasks that develop their knowledge and understanding (e.g., listening to succinct explanations, observing relevant demonstrations, answering focused questions) and that enhance their planning and evaluating skills (e.g., making decisions about how to link movements within a sequence, providing constructive feedback to a partner).

Assessment of pupils' knowledge and understanding should be through practically applied tasks (e.g., performing part of a warm-up, umpiring or refereeing a game, performing exercises to strengthen or stretch particular muscles).

Some non-active tasks (e.g., finding out about activity opportunities in the local community) can be given as physical education homework (i.e., preparation for subsequent PE lessons) or incorporated within related curriculum areas (e.g., PSHE).

developmentally appropriate physical education programme accommodates every child, from the physically gifted to the physically challenged, and takes into account a variety of individual characteristics such as stage of development; previous movement experiences; and activity, fitness and skill levels.

Teachers should not expect all children in a class to perform the same exercise in the same way for the same amount of time. This is unreasonable given the differences in maturation among pupils of the same age (figure 3.2). Differentiation is a key concept in effective teaching and learning and involves planned interventions by the teacher with the intention of maximising the achievements of pupils based on their differing needs. Such planned interventions can include several variations:

- Tasks—presenting tasks with different degrees of difficulty
- Outcome or response—permitting a range of responses, allowing pupils to work at different paces
- Support—providing extra attention or resources, providing additional encouragement
- Resources—using equipment that is easier or more challenging, altering the size of the playing area, ensuring that worksheets can be understood by all
- Group structure—permitting small-group work, providing individual tutoring, selecting mixed ability or setting as appropriate.

Commitment and effort to improve should be encouraged through praise. To promote participation, teachers must reward effort and personal progress and not focus predominantly or solely on performance.

WHAT IS 'INCLUSIVE' PHYSICAL ACTIVITY?

To promote current and future involvement in physical activity effectively, exercise experiences should be offered that meet individual needs and preferences. In practising and promoting the principle of equity, it is necessary to integrate all pupils including the least active, least competent and those with learning, physical or sensory impairments or specific health conditions.

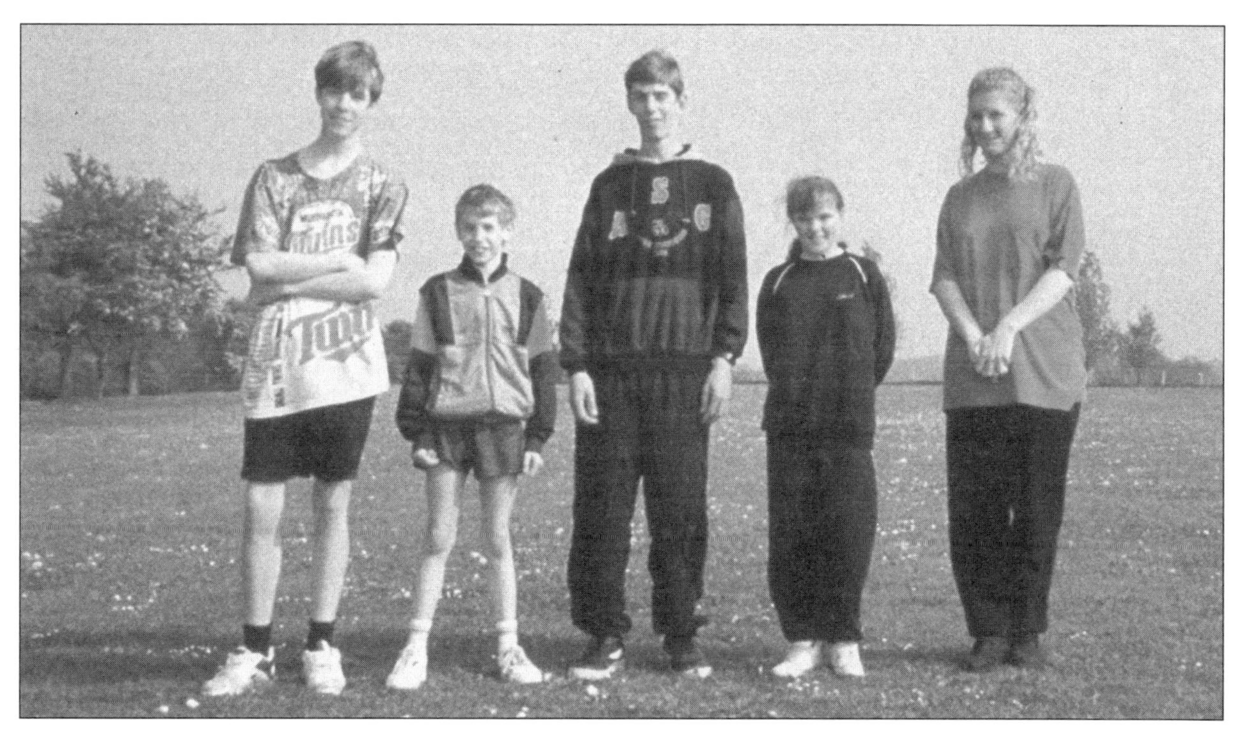

Figure 3.2 Pupils of the same age can vary in height, shape and weight.

Often, the main barrier to participation in physical activity is not a specific medical condition or impairment but the attitudinal, economic and environmental barriers that society places in the way. For young people to have increased access to physical activity, it is necessary to change the activity environment, such as improving teachers' ability to adopt more flexible approaches to the delivery of physical education. Every effort must be made to explore ways of including, rather than excluding, young people. This might involve consultation with the young people and their parents, carers and therapists.

Teachers need to select teaching approaches that ensure inclusion and permit every child to be actively involved. This avoids focusing on the specific impairments of young people and concentrates instead on changes to the activity to make it more accessible to a range of abilities. Teachers can extend tasks and make meaningful modifications to provide an inclusive challenge for all young people. Successful participation at an early stage in the introduction of an activity is a key factor in developing confidence and maintaining enthusiasm. Imagination on the part of the teacher and application by the young person can usually overcome any inability to perform a specific skill or action.

Examples of approaches that teachers can use to involve a wide range of abilities include the following:

- Inclusive activities—everyone is included without adaptation or modification. This is particularly possible during warm-ups and cool-downs and in circuit activities in which individuals are permitted to work at their level.
- Modified activities—changes to the rules, area or equipment used can facilitate inclusion (e.g., reducing the distance that some individuals travel, some players have more 'lives').
- Parallel activities—all take part in the same activity but in different ways (e.g., players in ability-matched games or zones, players are given specific roles such as shooter or goalkeeper, some participate from a seated position whilst others stand).
- Included activities—both disabled and non-disabled young people participate in adapted versions of an activity specifically designed for young disabled people (e.g., chair-based exercises, table-top games, seated volleyball).

- Separate activities—young disabled people practise an activity on their own or with disabled peers (e.g., practising a wheelchair routine to music, practising for a local disability event).

The vast majority of disabled and non-disabled young people can participate in health-related activities with little or no adaptation. Certain medical considerations, however, may preclude some young disabled people from participating in specific exercises. It is important to check with support staff, parents, carers and the young people themselves before they participate.

Strategies for adapting activities to facilitate inclusion include the following:

- In situations in which a young person cannot participate in a particular exercise or activity, provide a positive alternative rather than excluding an individual (e.g., offer a different or alternative version of an exercise). It is always possible to provide a positive alternative.
- If uncertain about an individual's exercise tolerance or fitness capability, alternate passive and active phases or build in frequent rest periods until this is established. Provide alternatives that enable individuals to reduce the intensity of an exercise (e.g., some can choose to walk or travel slowly between activities rather than run or move quickly).
- Abstract concepts such as weight transference or 'feeling a stretch' may not be within the experience of some young people. Provide clear visual demonstrations or find a way of isolating the desired movement (e.g., stretch with the support of the floor rather than standing).
- Offer non-weight-bearing alternatives or reduced resistance, especially during individuals' early experiences of exercises.
- Think about communicating ideas in the way most appropriate to the individual (e.g., permitting a visually impaired young person to 'feel' a movement through manual guidance such as holding a teacher's arm whilst the teacher performs an arm movement).

Other strategies to maximise involvement include changes to any of the following:

- Size of the area (ex.g., increasing it to allow more reaction time or reducing it to minimise travelling distance)
- Equipment (e.g., changing the size, shape, density or colour of a ball to improve catching skills)
- Number of participants (e.g., reducing the number of players in a small-sided game to increase everyone's involvement)
- Task (e.g., giving specific roles to some individuals)
- Time taken to complete the task (e.g., allowing some individuals more time)
- Interpretations of the skill requirements (e.g., 'receiving' or 'gathering' can be encouraged in place of 'catching'; transferring weight, mobility or wheelchair skills can be encouraged in place of 'running, jumping or hopping')
- Body position (e.g., changing the angle of a chair or wheelchair to provide a better position)

HOW CAN PUPIL PROGRESS BE ASSESSED IN HRE?

Achievement in HRE relates to improvements in the following:

- Knowledge and understanding
- Competence and motor skills

» Behavioural skills
» Attitudes and confidence

These improvements can be monitored in several ways:

» Responses to focused questions (pupil-teacher or pupil-pupil) and practical tasks
» Teacher observation of pupil performance in practical tasks
» Pupils taking more responsibility for their actions within and outside lessons
» Pupils' attendance, participation and commitment in physical education lessons
» Pupils' participation and commitment in extra-curricular activities
» Pupils' participation in physical activity outside of school

The following examples illustrate these strategies. Some are pertinent to particular key stages (KS):

» Pupil answers (pupil-pupil or pupil-teacher) to focused questions:

 How do you feel when you are active? (KS 1)

 What happens to your breathing when you exercise? (KS 1)

 Why does your heart rate change when you exercise? (KS 2)

 Which muscles are working hard when you run? (KS 2 or 3)

 Why is it important to stretch muscles after you have worked them? (KS 2 or 3)

 How much activity is recommended for young people? (KS 3)

 Explain how stronger upper-body muscles help you throw farther. (KS 4)

 What are some of the main reasons why young people are not active? (KS 4)

» Pupil responses to the following tasks:

 Show me an exercise that makes your heart pump quicker. (KS 1 or 2)

 Show me a stretch for the muscles in the back of your leg. (KS 2 or 3)

 Perform an exercise that will strengthen your abdominal muscles. (KS 3)

 For next week's lesson, make a list of the different places in the local area where you could be active (other than at school). (KS 3)

» Pupil entries in activity diaries (e.g., keeping a record for a number of weeks of all the activity, sport, dance and exercise performed at school, home, travelling and in the local area)
» The proportion of physical education lessons missed or not participated in by a pupil
» The degree of interest shown and effort put into physical education lessons
» Pupil involvement in school clubs, practices and events
» Pupil involvement in out-of-school clubs, activities and events.

Assessment of pupil achievement can be formative (ongoing) or summative (at the end of a unit). Formative methods help ensure that assessment is integral to teaching and learning (rather than a tagged-on addition).

To monitor long-term participation, it would be interesting and desirable to have information about young peoples' participation in physical activity after they leave primary or secondary school. For example, how many primary school pupils drop out of voluntary physical activity when they move to secondary school? What proportion of teenage girls give up exercise when they leave secondary school? Although it may be unrealistic for teachers to compile this information regularly, others might collect it, perhaps a teacher-researcher (as part of a further degree or

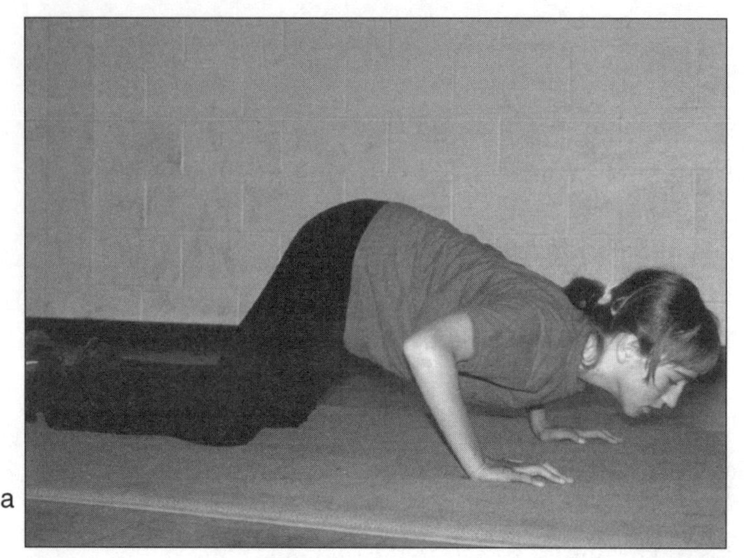
a

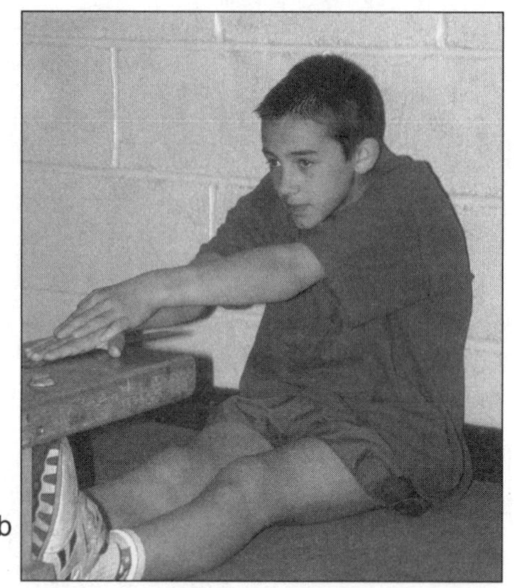
b

Figure 3.3 Two tests that can be used to assess pupils' muscular fitness are *(a)* push-ups and *(b)* the sit and reach.

special area of interest), an examination student (a pupil following an 'A' level course in physical education or sport studies) or an outside research group (health promotion unit or students from a local college or university).

Teachers will inevitably pick up information informally about their ex-pupils' involvement in local sports clubs and exercise classes. This can provide some feedback about the impact of the physical education programme on their long-term participation. It is recognised, however, that a multitude of factors influence activity patterns (e.g., the transition from school to work; competing activities such as homework, helping around the home, going to discos or clubs). The school curriculum can help prepare pupils for such transitions so that physical activity remains a valued aspect of their lives.

A commonly employed monitoring method in health-related programmes is fitness testing (figure 3.3). For a number of reasons, however, fitness testing is a controversial issue in educational settings. The following section helps to explain the issues associated with fitness testing and makes recommendations for primary and secondary school teachers.

FITNESS TESTING: TO TEST OR NOT TO TEST?

Much debate has occurred about the educational value of fitness testing in the physical education curriculum. The following is a summary of the main issues associated with fitness testing and some recommendations are presented in box 3.3.

What Purpose Do Fitness Tests Serve?

Fitness tests can provide a measure of pupils' fitness in a range of components (e.g., stamina, strength, flexibility) and can motivate pupils to increase their activity and fitness levels. Fitness tests may also be demeaning, embarrassing and uncomfortable for at-risk sedentary children and can be a negative experience that turns some children off rather than on to exercise.

What Do Fitness Tests Measure?

Fitness tests can provide pupils with a measure of the components of fitness. But fitness tests may also provide relatively crude measures and may be low in

Box 3.3
Recommendations

- Present fitness testing in a positive and individualised manner that promotes learning and provides pupils with personalised baseline scores from which to improve their activity and fitness levels.
- Ensure that testing is child centred and developmentally appropriate. It is important to focus on personal improvement over time, not on comparisons among pupils (e.g., averages, norms, percentiles).
- Ensure that health-related learning concepts are delivered during the fitness testing process (e.g., explaining the relevance of each fitness component and ensuring that pupils understand how to go about improving each component).
- Aim to make testing a positive experience. Avoid compulsory use of exhausting maximal tests. Minimise the public nature of testing, ensure prior practice and aim to provide personalised feedback.
- Do not assume that fitness testing will increase pupils' activity levels. Adopt activity promotion measures (e.g., monitoring and encouraging activity) and ensure that all pupils know of and have access to activity opportunities.
- Fitness testing can be part of but should not dominate a HRE programme. Ensure that pupils understand its relevance and focus on the process of being active more than the result of being fit.
- Monitor health-related components of fitness and use developmentally appropriate exercises (e.g., lower-level versions of exercises). Avoid or modify tests designed for adults and use sub-maximal tests. If choosing to measure body composition, do so sensitively and as privately as possible.

validity and reliability. Fitness tests may merely highlight different levels of maturation.

What Do Pupils Learn From Fitness Tests?

Pupils can learn about the various components of fitness, their relevance to everyday life, health and sport performance, and ways to assess their fitness and monitor it over time in a range of components. But fitness tests may be delivered with minimal planned learning, little follow-up guidance and limited pupil understanding of why they perform fitness tests, what the results indicate, and how they should respond to the results.

What Are Pupils' Views About Fitness Testing?

Children can enjoy fitness testing and be motivated by it to be more active and to improve their fitness. Research indicates, however, that some children view fitness tests as painful, negative experiences and may even try to avoid them.

Does Fitness Testing Increase Activity Levels?

Fitness testing may motivate some pupils to be more active. But little evidence exists that fitness testing increases activity levels. Indeed, it is possible that fitness tests demotivate children with low levels of fitness.

How Prevalent Are Fitness Tests?

Sixty percent of secondary schools include fitness testing in the PE curriculum (usually compulsory for the lower age ranges). The testing of fitness as a product can dominate HRE programmes and detract from promoting the process of being more active.

What Types of Fitness Tests Are Being Used?

A range of maximal (e.g., timed distance run, bleep test) and sub-maximal (e.g., step test) fitness tests are available to measure both health-related (stamina, strength, flexibility, body composition) and skill-related components of physical fitness (agility, balance, co-ordination, reaction time, power, speed). Some teachers, however, use developmentally inappropriate procedures such as adult exercises (e.g., full push-ups) and maximal tests designed for use with elite adult sportspeople. Many pupils dislike and are turned off by exhausting and painful forms of exercise.

SUMMARY

Formal fitness testing of primary school children is not recommended. It is neither necessary nor appropriate because of the early maturational stage of pupils and the limited evidence that younger children readily show fitness gains following exercise programmes. It is desirable, however, for primary school children to be involved in simple monitoring methods such as recording some effects of exercise on their bodies (e.g., changes in heart rate, breathing rate, temperature, appearance, feelings) and keeping activity diaries over a short period.

Fitness testing of secondary school children is acceptable but not essential. If included, it should occur as part of a planned programme of study that focuses on helping young people understand the effects and benefits of exercise and increasing their activity levels. It should not be allowed to dominate a health-related programme of study. Administering fitness tests to acquire data for records, without attention to the tests' educational role, is not advised.

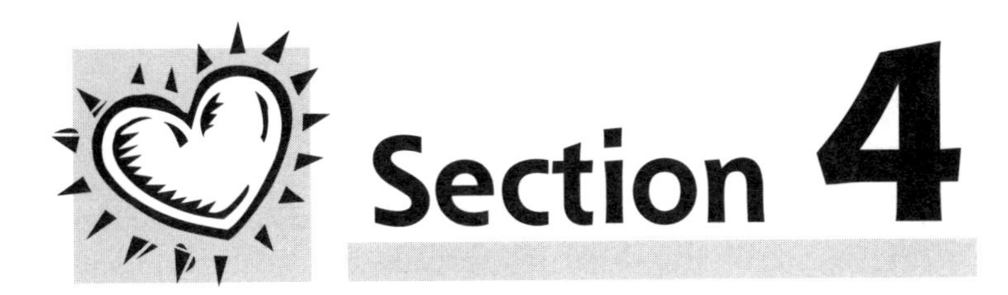

Section 4

Requirements and Approaches

NATIONAL CURRICULUM FOR PHYSICAL EDUCATION IN ENGLAND

The programmes of study within the National Curriculum for Physical Education in England set out what pupils should be taught, and the attainment target sets out the expected standards of pupils' performance. Schools choose how to organise their school curriculum to include the programmes of study for physical education.

The government believes that two hours of physical activity a week, including the National Curriculum for Physical Education and extra-curricular activities, should be an aspiration for all schools. This applies throughout all key stages.

The programmes of study provide the basis for planning schemes of work. When planning, consideration should be given to the general teaching requirements for inclusion, use of language, use of information and communication technology, and health and safety. Within the National Curriculum for Physical Education in England, examples are provided of ways in which the teaching of physical education can contribute to learning across the curriculum (e.g., spiritual, moral, social and cultural development; key skills in communication, application of number, information technology, working with others, improving own learning and performance, problem-solving; thinking skills, work-related learning, and education for sustainable development). The National Curriculum for Physical Education in England identifies the following aspects of physical education in which pupils make progress:

- Acquiring and developing skills
- Selecting and applying skills, tactics and compositional ideas
- Evaluating and improving performance
- Knowledge and understanding of fitness and health

When evaluating and improving performance, teaching should make connections between developing, selecting and applying skills, tactics and compositional ideas, and fitness and health.

NATIONAL CURRICULUM FOR PHYSICAL EDUCATION IN WALES

The programmes of study within the National Curriculum for Physical Education in Wales set out what to teach to the majority of pupils in each key stage. Teachers should provide opportunities, where appropriate, for pupils to develop and apply the following common requirements through their study of physical education: knowledge and understanding of the characteristics of Wales, communication skills, mathematical skills, information technology skills, problem-solving skills, creative skills, and personal and social education. The National Curriculum for Physical Education in Wales states that **health-related exercise** should be taught at each key stage. One of the four areas of experience within the key stage 4 programme of study is **exercise activities** (non-competitive forms of exercise, such as step aerobics, jogging, weight-training, cycling, circuit-training and skipping).

HRE Within the Key Stage Focus Statements of the National Curriculum for Physical Education

The following table summarizes the key stage focus statements for each country.

Key stage	England	Wales
1	Pupils build on their natural enthusiasm for movement, using it to explore and learn about their world.	Activities should build on pupils' enthusiasm and energy for movement and play using indoor and outdoor environments.
2	Pupils enjoy being active and using their creativity and imagination in physical activity. They develop an understanding of how to succeed in different activities and learn how to evaluate and recognise their success.	Pupils should be taught to persevere longer at improving and adapting skills, showing that they can sustain activity for increasingly longer periods.
3	Pupils start to identify the types of activity they prefer to be involved with.	Pupils should be taught to exercise safely and appreciate the value of regular exercise.
4	Pupils decide whether to get involved in physical activity that focuses mainly on competing or performing, promoting health and well-being, or developing personal fitness. The view they have of their skillfulness and physical competence gives them the confidence to become involved in exercise and activity out of school and in later life.	Selected activities should take account of previous achievement, personal interest and levels of pupil motivation. Through physical activity, pupils should be helped to acquire confidence, self-esteem, respect for themselves and others and to develop a commitment to an active lifestyle. They should be taught to plan, perform, monitor and evaluate a safe and effective health-related exercise programme that meets their personal needs and preferences.

HRE Within the Attainment Target for Physical Education

The following table details HRE elements from the level descriptions composing the attainment target within the National Curriculum for Physical Education (NCPE) in England and Wales. The attainment target describes the types and range of performance (including exceptional) that pupils working at that level should characteristically demonstrate. In deciding on a pupil's level of attainment at the end of a key stage, teachers should judge which description best fits the pupil's performance.

Level	Key stage	NCPE for England	NCPE for Wales
1	1	Pupils talk about how to exercise safely and how their bodies feel during an activity.	Pupils recognise and name body parts used in movement and balance, simple games and basic actions. They describe what they are doing or how they feel. They show increasing awareness of the space away from others in which to work safely.
2	1, 2 (expected attainment of majority of pupils aged 7)	Pupils understand how to exercise safely and describe how their bodies feel during different activities.	Pupils show sufficient control to work safely with others when using games equipment and gymnastics apparatus and take some responsibility for taking them out and putting them away. They recognise and describe the changes that happen to their bodies during exercise.
3	2, 3	Pupils give reasons why warming up before an activity is important and why physical activity is good for health.	Pupils provide simple explanations for the changes that take place in their bodies during exercise.
4	1, 2, 3 (expected attainment of majority of pupils aged 11)	Pupils explain and apply basic safety principles in preparing for exercise. They describe what effects exercise has on their bodies and how it is valuable to their fitness and health.	Pupils explain reasons for the short-term effects of exercise on the body and show some understanding of the importance of exercise to aspects of a healthy lifestyle.
5	1, 2, 3 (level 5 or 6: expected attainment of majority of pupils aged 14)	Pupils explain how the body reacts during different types of exercise, and they warm up and cool down in ways that suit the activity. They explain why regular, safe exercise is good for their fitness and health.	Pupils perform relevant and safe warm-up and cool-down routines and begin to take some responsibility for their planning. They know how to monitor a range of short-term effects on the cardiovascular system and show some understanding of the value of exercise to social and psychological well-being.
6	3 (level 5 or 6: expected attainment of majority of pupils aged 14)	Pupils explain how to prepare for, and recover from, the activities. They explain how different types of exercise contribute to their fitness and health and describe how they might get involved in other types of activities and exercise.	Pupils take increasing responsibility for the planning and execution of safe exercises, know which exercises to avoid to prevent possible injury, and understand that appropriate training can improve fitness and performance. They understand many of the

(continued)

HRE Within the Attainment Target for Physical Education *(continued)*

Level	Key stage	NCPE for England	NCPE for Wales
			long-term effects of exercise on physical, mental and social health.
7	3	Pupils explain the principles of practice and training and apply them effectively. They explain the benefits of regular, planned activity on health and fitness and plan their own appropriate exercise and activity programme.	Pupils understand the long-term effects of exercise on physical, mental and social health.
8	3 (very able pupils)	Pupils use their knowledge of health and fitness to plan and evaluate their own and others' exercise and activity programmes.	Pupils consider factors affecting participation in physical activity from different perspectives.
Exceptional performance	3 (exceptional pupils)	Pupils consistently apply appropriate knowledge and understanding of health and fitness in all aspects of their work.	Pupils understand that appropriate training can improve fitness and performance, and they appreciate the value of exercise to social and psychological well-being. They use the technical vocabulary of physical education and health-related exercise consistently and accurately to explain factors affecting participation in physical activity.

HRE Within the National Curriculum for England

The following table details health-related exercise and associated requirements within physical education; personal, social and health education (PSHE) and citizenship; and science.

Physical education	PSHE and citizenship	Science
KEY STAGE 1 **Pupils should be taught the following:** • To understand how important it is to be active • To recognise and describe how their bodies feel during different activities	**Pupils should be taught the following:** • To recognise what they like and dislike, what is fair and unfair and what is right and wrong • To think about themselves, learn from their experiences and recognise what they are good at • To make simple choices that affect their health and well-being • To maintain personal hygiene • To know the names of the main parts of the body • To know rules for, and ways of, keeping safe, including basic road	**Pupils should be taught the following:** • To recognise and compare the main external parts of the bodies of humans and other animals • To know that humans and other animals need food and water to stay alive • To understand that exercising and eating the right types and amounts of food helps to keep humans healthy

Physical education	PSHE and citizenship	Science
	safety, and about people who can help them to stay safe • To listen to other people and play and work cooperatively	
KEY STAGE 2 **Pupils should be taught the following:** • How exercise affects the body in the short term • How to warm up and prepare appropriately for different activities • Why physical activity is good for their health and well-being • Why wearing appropriate clothing and being hygienic are good for their health and safety	**Pupils should be taught the following:** • To recognise their worth as individuals by identifying positive things about themselves and their achievements, seeing their mistakes, making amends and setting personal goals • To understand what makes a healthy lifestyle, including the benefits of exercise and healthy eating, what affects mental health and how to make informed choices • To recognise the different risks in different situations and then decide how to behave responsibly, including sensible road use and judging what kind of physical contact is acceptable or unacceptable • To know school rules about health and safety, basic emergency aid procedures and where to get help	**Pupils should be taught the following:** • That the body needs food for activity and growth and that an adequate and varied diet is important for health • That the heart acts as a pump to circulate the blood through vessels around the body, including through the lungs • That exercise and rest affect pulse rate • That humans and some other animals have skeletons and muscles to support and protect their bodies and to help them move • That tobacco, alcohol and other drugs affect the human body and personal health • That exercise is important for good health
KEY STAGE 3 **Pupils should be taught the following:** • How to prepare for and recover from specific activities • How different types of activity affect specific aspects of their fitness • How regular exercise and good hygiene improve health • How to become involved in activities that are good for their personal and social health and well-being	**Pupils should be taught the following:** • To reflect on and assess their strengths in relation to personality, work and leisure • To know how to keep healthy and what influences health, including the media • To understand that good relationships and an appropriate balance among work, leisure and exercise can promote physical and mental health • To recognise and manage risk and make safer choices about healthy lifestyles, different environments and travel	**Pupils should be taught the following:** • That the body needs a balanced diet containing carbohydrates, proteins, fats, minerals, vitamins, fibre and water and, that various foods are sources of these • That food is used as a fuel during respiration to maintain the body's activity and as a raw material for growth and repair • That the skeleton and joints have important roles and that antagonistic muscle pairs (e.g., biceps and triceps) create movement

(continued)

Physical education	PSHE and citizenship	Science
	• To know basic emergency aid procedures and where to get help and support	• That aerobic respiration involves a reaction in cells between oxygen and food in which glucose is broken down into carbon dioxide and water • That the abuse of alcohol, solvents and other drugs affects health
KEY STAGE 4 **Pupils should be taught the following:** • How preparation, training and fitness relate to and affect performance • How to design and carry out activity and training programmes that have specific purposes • How exercise and activity will improve personal, social and mental health and well-being • How to monitor and develop their own training, exercise and activity programmes in and out of school	**Pupils should be taught the following:** • To be aware of and assess their personal qualities, skills, achievements and potential so that they can set personal goals • To think about the alternatives and long- and short-term consequences when making decisions about personal health • To understand the link between eating patterns and self-image, including eating disorders • To seek professional advice confidently and find information about health • To recognise and follow health and safety requirements and develop the skills to cope with emergency situations that require basic aid procedures, including resuscitation techniques	**Pupils should be taught the following:** • How the processes of digestion work, including the function of organs and the role of enzymes, stomach acid and bile • How blood functions and what it is composed of • How the reflex arc makes rapid response to a stimulus possible • How humans maintain a constant body temperature • How the defence mechanisms of the body function, including the role of the skin and blood • How solvents, alcohol, tobacco and other drugs affect body functions

HRE Within the National Curriculum for Wales

The following table details health-related exercise and associated requirements within physical education, personal and social education (PSE), and science.

Physical education	Personal and social education	Science
KEY STAGE 1 **Throughout the key stage, pupils should be taught the following:** • To understand the changes that happen to their bodies as they exercise and to recognise the effects	**PSE provision should enable pupils to do the following:** • Have respect for their bodies and those of others	**Pupils should be taught the following:** • The names of the main external parts (e.g., hand, elbow, knee) of the human body

Physical education	Personal and social education	Science
• To describe changes to their breathing (faster), heart rate (heart pumps more quickly), appearance (feel and look hotter) and feelings (tired or more energetic) • To adopt good posture when sitting, standing and taking part in activity • To prepare for and recover from activity appropriately • To understand that the body uses food and drink to release energy for exercise • To know that regular exercise improves health and how one feels • To recognise that exercise helps body parts work well Pupils should be taught to wear appropriate clothing and footwear for different activities and to remove jewellery that might cause injury.	• Value being healthy and be positive about the actions necessary to be healthy • Begin to take responsibility for their actions • Feel positive about themselves • Practise making informed decisions • Develop everyday practical skills **Pupils should know the following:** • That exercise and hygiene and the right types and amount of food are important to keep their bodies healthy • What is fair and unfair and what they believe to be right and wrong • What they are good at • How they can improve their learning	• That animals, including humans, move, need food and water, grow and reproduce • That exercising and eating the right types and amounts of food help humans to stay healthy
KEY STAGE 2 **Throughout the key stage, pupils should be taught the following:** • To sustain activity over appropriate periods in a range of physical activities (e.g., contrasting the demands of a walk to those of a longer run, different types of games, a long swim and a short dance) • To understand the short-term effects of exercise on the body (e.g., increased heart rate allows more oxygen to be delivered to the muscles; the heat produced is transferred to the body's surface [skin] so that body temperature stays normal) • To adopt good posture when sitting, standing and taking part in activity • To prepare for and recover from activity appropriately • To understand that the body needs a certain amount of energy for activity and that if more food and drink is taken in than is needed for activity body fat increases • To understand that exercise strengthens bones and muscles	**PSE provision should enable pupils to do the following:** • Have respect for their bodies and those of others and enjoy and take more responsibility for keeping the body safe and healthy • Take increasing responsibility for their actions • Feel positive about themselves and be confident in their own values • Develop decision-making skills • Develop practical skills necessary for everyday life **Pupils should know the following:** • The benefits of exercise and hygiene and the need for a variety of food for growth and activity • How to be safe at home, on the road, near water and in the sun	**Pupils should be taught the following:** • That the body needs different foods for activity and for growth • That an adequate and varied diet is needed to keep healthy • That the heart acts as a pump • That blood circulates in the body through arteries and veins • That the pulse gives a measure of the heart beat rate • That exercise and rest affect pulse rate • That humans and some other animals have skeletons and muscles to support and protect their bodies and to help them move • That tobacco, alcohol and other drugs can have harmful effects

(continued)

Physical education	Personal and social education	Science
• To recognise that exercise can be fun and sociable • To know that opportunities for exercise should be taken every day for it to be beneficial Throughout the key stage, pupils should be taught to recognise and follow relevant rules and safety procedures that apply in the different activities. They should be taught to wear appropriate clothing and footwear for different physical activities and to remove jewellery that might cause injury.	• Their strengths, weaknesses and targets for improvement • The ways in which they learn best	
KEY STAGE 3 **Throughout the key stage, pupils should be taught the following:** • To monitor a range of short-term effects on the cardiovascular system (e.g., changes in heart rate) and the musculo-skeletal system (e.g., changes in muscular strength, endurance and flexibility; improved muscle tone) • To appreciate the long-term effects of exercise on physical health (e.g., reduced risk of heart disease, osteoporosis, obesity; improved management of health conditions such as asthma) • To adopt good posture when sitting, standing and taking part in activity • To use relevant and safe warm-up and cool-down routines (e.g., mobility exercises, whole-body activities and static stretches) and to take responsibility for their planning and execution • To understand the differences between whole-body activities that help to reduce body fat and conditioning exercises that improve muscle tone • To realise that appropriate training can improve fitness and performance • To know the value of exercise to social and psychological well-being (e.g., increased confidence and self-esteem, decreased anxiety and stress) • To know the range of activity opportunities at school, home and in the local community and ways of incorporating exercise into their lifestyles (e.g., walking or cycling to school or to meet friends)	**PSE provision should enable pupils to do the following:** • Have a responsible attitude towards keeping the body safe and healthy • Take increasing responsibility for their actions • Value their achievements and success and be committed to lifelong learning in a changing world • Be disciplined and take responsibility for actions and decisions • Make decisions and choices effectively • Develop action plans and set targets • Review and reflect on learning and analyse strengths and weaknesses • Make reasoned judgements • Administer basic first aid **Pupils should know the following:** • The relationship between diet and good health and the importance of food safety • That maintaining regular exercise can have both mental and physical benefits • How to use their preferred learning styles to improve learning performance	**Pupils should be taught the following:** • That food is used as a fuel during respiration to maintain the body's activity and as a raw material for growth and repair • That the skeleton, joints and muscles have important roles in movement • That antagonistic muscle pairs (e.g., biceps and triceps) create movement • That aerobic respiration is a reaction in cells in which glucose reacts with oxygen and is broken down into carbon dioxide and water • That aerobic respiration provides energy for use by the body • That the abuse of alcohol, solvents and other drugs affects health

Physical education	Personal and social education	Science
Pupils should adopt safe practices and procedures when taking part in physical activities that might require the wearing of protective clothing, the removal of jewellery to avoid injury, the supervised use of equipment or response to specific weather conditions.	• How to manage time and organise themselves effectively	
KEY STAGE 4 **Throughout the key stage, pupils should be taught the following:** • To plan, perform, monitor and evaluate a safe and effective health-related exercise programme that meets their personal needs and preferences over an extended period • To know and be able to demonstrate a practical understanding of the key principles of exercise programming and training, including progression, overload, specificity, balance/moderation/variety, maintenance and reversibility **During this stage, pupils should have opportunities to do the following:** • Explore how to overcome constraints to being active and gain access to activity opportunities both in school and in the local community • Appreciate the exercise effects, health benefits and safety issues associated with their selected activities in the key stage 4 programme • Appreciate the risks associated with a sedentary lifestyle and with excessive forms and amounts of exercise	**PSE provision should enable pupils to do the following:** • Take responsibility for keeping the body safe and healthy and have a responsible attitude towards sexual relationships • Value their achievements and success and be committed to lifelong learning • Be disciplined and take responsibility for actions and decisions • Make decisions and choices effectively • Use relaxation, exercise and other techniques to manage stress • Review learning and performance, develop action plans and set targets • Make reasoned judgements • Administer basic first aid **Pupils should know the following:** • How to analyse and evaluate dietary information • That maintaining regular exercise can have both mental and physical benefits • The causes and effects of stress and the ways in which it can be managed • How to review their learning and set priorities for development and targets for improvement	**Pupils should be taught the following:** • How the processes of digestion work, including the role of enzymes, stomach acid and bile • How blood functions and what it is composed of • How the reflex arc, which involves a nerve impulse carried by neurons across synapses, makes rapid response to a stimulus possible • How humans maintain a constant body temperature • How the defence mechanisms of the body function, including the role of the skin and blood

Health-Related Exercise Learning Outcomes

This section presents an interpretation of the HRE requirements of the national curriculum for England and for Wales. The interpretation is expressed in the form of learning outcomes for each key stage that address the HRE requirements of the physical education curriculum and incorporate links with relevant health-related aspects of other subjects such as science and personal and social education. To make clear the range of coverage and the progression between key stages, the learning outcomes have been placed into four categories: safety issues, exercise effects, health benefits and activity promotion.

Safety issues	Exercise effects	Health benefits	Activity promotion
KEY STAGE 1 **PUPILS SHOULD ACHIEVE THESE LEARNING OUTCOMES:**			
a. Know and adhere to safety rules and practices (e.g., changing clothes for PE lessons, tying long hair back, removing jewellery, sitting and standing with good posture, wearing footwear when skipping with a rope, no running fast to touch walls) b. Know that activity starts with a gentle warm-up and finishes with a calming cool-down	a. Experience, recognise and describe the effects of exercise, including changes to the following: i. Breathing (e.g., becomes faster and deeper) ii. Heart rate (e.g., heart pumps more quickly) iii. Temperature (e.g., feel hotter) iv. Appearance (e.g., look hotter) v. Feelings (e.g., feeling good, more energetic, tired) vi. External body parts (e.g., arm and leg muscles are working) b. Know that the body uses food and drink to release energy for exercise	a. Know that regular exercise improves health in these ways: i. Makes you feel good (e.g., happy, pleased, content) ii. Helps body parts (e.g., bones and muscles) grow, develop and work well	a. Know when, where and how they can be active at school (in and out of lessons) b. Use opportunities to be active including playtimes
KEY STAGE 2 **PUPILS SHOULD ACHIEVE THESE LEARNING OUTCOMES:**			
a. Understand the need for safety rules and practices (e.g., adopting good posture at all times, being hygienic, changing clothes and having a wash after energetic activity, wearing footwear for some activities, following rules, protecting against cold weather,	a. Experience and understand the short-term effects of exercise: i. Increase in the rate and depth of breathing to provide more oxygen to the working muscles ii. Increase in the heart rate to pump more oxygen to the working muscles	a. Know that exercise strengthens bones and muscles (including the heart) and keeps joints flexible b. Know that exercise can help you to feel good about yourself and can be fun and sociable (e.g., involves sharing experiences and co-operating with others)	a. Be aware of their current levels of activity (e.g., daily, twice a week) b. Know when, where and how they can be active in school and outside c. Be able to make decisions about which physical activities they enjoy and know that individuals have different feelings

avoiding sunburn in hot weather, lifting safely, using space sensibly) b. Know the purpose of a warm-up and cool-down and recognise and describe parts of a warm-up and cool-down (i.e., exercises for the joints [e.g., arm circles], whole-body activities [e.g., jogging, skipping without a rope] and stretches for the whole body such as reaching long and tall or parts of the body such as the lower leg or calf muscles)	iii. Increase in the temperature because working muscles produce energy as heat and the skin becomes moist, sticky and sweaty because the heat produced by the muscles is transferred to the body's surface (skin) to control body temperature iv. Flushed appearance likely because blood vessels become wider and closer to the surface of the skin v. Varied feelings and moods (e.g., having fun and being with friends) b. Know that the body needs a certain amount of energy every day in the form of food and drink to function properly (e.g., for normal growth, development and daily living) and that body fat increases if more food and drink is taken in than is needed (e.g., for breathing, growing, sleeping, eating, moving, exercise)	c. Know that regular exercise permits daily activities to be performed more easily d. Know that being active helps maintain a healthy body weight	about the types and amounts of exercise they choose to do d. Use opportunities to be active for 30 to 60 minutes every day (with rest periods as necessary), including lessons, playtimes and club activities
KEY STAGE 3 **PUPILS SHOULD ACHIEVE THESE LEARNING OUTCOMES:**			
a. Demonstrate understanding of safe exercise practices (e.g., tying long hair back and removing jewellery to avoid injury; adopting good posture when sitting, standing and moving; performing exercises with good technique; washing or showering following energetic activity; using equipment and facilities with permission and, where necessary, under supervision;	a. Understand and monitor a range of short-term effects of exercise on these body systems: i. Cardiovascular system (e.g., changes in breathing and heart rate, temperature, appearance, feelings, recovery rate, ability to pace oneself and remain within a target zone) ii. Musculo-skeletal system (e.g., increases in muscular strength,	a. Know and understand a range of long-term benefits of exercise on physical health: i. Reduced risk of chronic disease (e.g., heart disease) ii. Reduced risk of bone disease (e.g., osteoporosis) iii. Reduced risk of some health conditions (e.g., obesity, back pain)	a. Be able to access information about a range of activity opportunities at school, home and in the local community and know ways of incorporating exercise into their lifestyles (e.g., walking or cycling to school or to meet friends, helping around the home or garden) b. Reflect on their activity strengths and preferences and know how to become involved in activities

(continued)

Safety issues	Exercise effects	Health benefits	Activity promotion
administering basic first aid; wearing adequate protection such as goalkeeping gloves and leg pads for certain activities; coping with specific weather conditions such as using sunscreen to avoid burning in the sun and drinking fluids to prevent dehydration; knowing procedures associated with specific activities) b. Demonstrate concern for and understanding of back care by lifting, carrying, placing and using equipment responsibly and with good technique c. Understand why certain exercises and practices are not recommended (e.g., standing toe touches, straight leg sit-ups, bouncing in stretches, flinging movements) and be able to perform safe alternatives (e.g., seated 'sit-and-reach' stretch, curl-ups with bent legs, holding stretches still, performing movements with control) d. Understand the value of preparing for and recovering from activity and the possible consequences of not doing so, and be able to explain the purpose of and plan and perform each component of a warm-up and cool-down (i.e., mobility exercises, whole-body activities, static stretches) for general activity (e.g., games, athletics) and for a specific activity (e.g., volleyball, high jump, circuit-training)	endurance and flexibility; improved muscle tone and posture; enhanced functional capacity and sport or dance performance) b. Know and understand that appropriate training can improve fitness and performance and that different types of activity affect specific aspects of fitness (e.g., running affects cardiovascular fitness) c. Understand the differences between whole-body activities (e.g., walking, jogging, cycling, dancing, swimming) that help reduce body fat and conditioning exercises (e.g., straight and twisting curl-ups) that improve muscle tone	iv. Improved management of some health conditions (e.g., asthma, diabetes, arthritis) b. Know and understand that exercise can enhance mental health and social and psychological well-being (e.g., enjoying being with friends, increased confidence and self-esteem, decreased anxiety and stress) and that an appropriate balance among work, leisure and exercise promotes good health c. Know and understand that increasing activity levels and eating a balanced diet can help maintain a healthy body weight (energy balance equation) but that the body needs a minimum daily energy intake to function properly and that strict dieting and excessive exercising can damage one's health d. Know and understand how each activity area (athletics, dance, games, gymnastics, OAA, swimming) can contribute to physical health and to social and psychological well-being (e.g., can improve stamina, assist weight management, strengthen bones, be enjoyable)	c. Participate in activity of at least moderate intensity for a minimum of half an hour and preferably for one hour every day (i.e., 30 to 60 minutes accumulated during a day) d. At least twice a week, participate in activities that help to enhance and maintain muscular strength and flexibility and bone health (e.g., dance, aerobics, skipping, games, body conditioning or resistance exercises) e. Be able to monitor and evaluate personal activity levels over a period (e.g., by keeping an activity diary for four to six weeks and reflecting on the experience)

e. Be able to perform with good technique developmentally appropriate cardiovascular activities and strength and flexibility exercises for each of the major muscle groups			
KEY STAGE 4 **PUPILS SHOULD ACHIEVE THESE LEARNING OUTCOMES:**			
a. Be able to recognise and manage risk and apply safe exercise principles and procedures (e.g., not exercising when unwell or injured; avoiding prolonged high-impact exercise; administering first aid, including resuscitation techniques; avoiding excessive amounts of exercise) b. Be able to evaluate warm-ups and cool-downs in terms of safety, effectiveness and relevance to the specific activity and take responsibility for their own safe and effective preparation for and recovery from activity c. Be able to select, perform and evaluate safe, effective and developmentally appropriate exercises from a range of lifetime activities (e.g., jogging, swimming, cycling, aerobics, step aerobics, circuit-training, weight-training)	a. Know and understand that training exercises and practices are specific to an activity and affect performance b. Know and understand that training programmes develop both health-related components (cardiovascular fitness, muscular strength and endurance, flexibility, body composition, composure, decision-making) and skill-related components of physical and mental fitness (agility, balance, co-ordination, power, reaction time, speed, concentration, determination)	a. Know and understand that frequent and appropriate exercise enhances the physical, social and psychological well-being of all individuals including the young and old, disabled and non-disabled, and those with health conditions (e.g., asthma, depression) and chronic disease (e.g., arthritis) b. Know that exercise can help manage stress and contribute to a happy, healthy and balanced lifestyle c. Appreciate the risks associated with a sedentary lifestyle and with excessive behaviour (e.g., developing eating disorders and over-exercising) d. Know and understand how each activity area (e.g., gymnastics, swimming, athletics) can contribute to specific components of health-related fitness (e.g., gymnastics involves weight-bearing actions and thus develops muscular strength and endurance)	a. Be able to plan, perform, monitor and evaluate a safe and effective health-related exercise programme that meets their personal needs and preferences over an extended period (e.g., over 6 to 12 weeks) b. Have access to physical activity personnel (e.g., sports development officers, school sport co-ordinators, coaches and instructors), facilities (e.g., sports, health and fitness clubs and leisure centres) and services (e.g., courses, projects, leaflets, pamphlets) within the local community c. Experience a range of lifetime physical activities (e.g., walking, jogging, swimming, cycling, aerobics, step aerobics, circuit-training, weight-training, skipping, aqua exercise) d. Know, understand and be able to demonstrate a practical understanding of the key principles of exercise programming and training, including the following: i. Progression (developing the amount of exercise by gradually increasing frequency, intensity or duration)

(continued)

Health-Related Exercise Learning Outcomes *(continued)*

Safety issues	**Exercise effects**	**Health benefits**	**Activity promotion**
			ii. Overload (progressively enabling the body to do more exercise than previously accustomed) iii. Specificity (a particular exercise or sporting activity benefits specific muscles, joints, bones, energy systems) iv. Balance, moderation and variety (maximising exercise benefits and minimising risks) v. Maintenance (establishing a routine, sustaining a commitment, coping with relapse) vi. Reversibility (the benefits of exercise are gradually lost after a break) vii. Cost-benefit ratio (weighing up the costs involved, such as time, money, transport and sweating, against the benefits, such as maintaining body weight, feeling good, improving fitness) e. Assess their qualities, skills, achievements and potential so that they can set personal goals that assist them in following the activity recommendations for young people and developing a commitment to an active lifestyle f. Be aware of factors affecting participation and constraints to being active and explore how to overcome the latter to gain access to and sustain involvement in activity

Approaches to HRE Within the National Curriculum

The teaching of HRE can be organised in several ways. Each approach has specific strengths and limitations. Curriculum leaders in physical education and heads of physical education departments are familiar with their own curriculum, colleagues, pupils and resources. They are therefore in a good position to make appropriate decisions concerning the approach or approaches adopted. These approaches may vary among schools. Teachers will make a decision by considering the strengths and limitations of each of the possible approaches (see table). The responsibility of teachers is to deliver the statutory requirements effectively to combat the trend towards sedentary living.

Approach	Strengths	Limitations
PERMEATION (INTEGRATION) An approach in which HRE is taught through the PE activity areas (i.e., through athletics, dance, games, gymnastics, outdoor and adventurous activities, and swimming).	HRE knowledge, understanding and skills can be seen as part of and integral to all PE experiences. Children learn that all physical activities can contribute towards good health and can become part of an active lifestyle.	HRE knowledge, understanding and skills may become lost or marginalised amongst other information relating to skills and performance; pupils may be overloaded with information; much liaison activity is required to ensure that all pupils receive similar information from different teachers; and the approach may be somewhat ad hoc and piecemeal.
FOCUSED (DISCRETE) An approach involving teaching HRE through specific focused units of work within either a PE or PSE-PSHE programme.	A specific focus can help ensure that HRE does not become lost or take second place to other information. HRE is less likely to be regarded as an assumed by-product of PE lessons, and HRE is perceived as important through having its own time slot and identity. The value and status of the associated knowledge, understanding and skills are raised.	HRE may be seen in isolation and not closely linked to the PE activity areas. The HRE knowledge, understanding and skills may be delivered over a period with long gaps in between, which is problematic in terms of cohesion and progression (e.g., one short unit per year). The knowledge base may be delivered in such a way as to reduce activity levels within PE lessons (e.g., too much teacher talk).
TOPIC An approach involving a series of lessons following a specific topic or theme that is taught through PE and classroom lessons. This may incorporate both permeation and focused units.	HRE may be delivered in a more holistic manner with closer links to other health behaviours (such as eating a balanced diet) and other national curriculum subjects. The area can be covered in more depth and be closely related to pupils' personal experiences. The amount of time engaged in physical activity in PE lessons might be increased if introductory and follow-up work is conducted in the classroom.	A topic or theme-based approach may be more time consuming with respect to planning. This approach could be less practically oriented than other approaches (if it incorporates a high degree of classroom based work).
COMBINED Any combination of permeation, focused and topic-based approaches is possible.	This builds on the strengths of each approach. It ensures that value is placed on HRE and that the area of work is closely linked to all PE experiences and other health behaviours and related subjects.	Combined approaches initially may be more time consuming to plan, structure, implement and coordinate within the curriculum.

Mapping HRE

The following is an example of how the teaching of HRE can be mapped at each key stage to ensure that the content and delivery are properly planned and structured. It also provides teachers with a coherent framework and ensures that pupils receive consistent and co-ordinated messages and experiences. For each key stage, teachers need to consider the variety of possible approaches and make decisions about how the learning is to be organised within their curriculum. The mapping tables permit the HRE learning outcomes for each key stage to be set within the areas of activity or within focused topics or units.

KEY STAGE 1

Area	**Safety issues**	**Exercise effects**	**Health benefits**	**Activity promotion**
Dance				
Games				
Gymnastics				
Swimming				
Topic approach				

KEY STAGE 2

Area	**Safety issues**	**Exercise effects**	**Health benefits**	**Activity promotion**
Athletics				
Dance				
Games				
Gymnastics				
OAA				
Swimming				
Topic approach or focused unit(s)				

KEY STAGE 3

Area	Safety issues	Exercise effects	Health benefits	Activity promotion
Athletics				
Dance				
Games				
Gymnastics				
OAA				
Swimming				
Focused unit(s)				
PSHE-PSE				

KEY STAGE 4

Area	Safety issues	Exercise effects	Health benefits	Activity promotion
Athletics				
Dance				
Games				
Gymnastics				
OAA				
Swimming				
*Sport**				
*Exercise activities**				

(continued)

Mapping HRE *(continued)*

Area	Safety issues	Exercise effects	Health benefits	Activity promotion
Focused unit(s)				
PSHE-PSE				

* Applies to the National Curriculum for Physical Education in Wales.
From *Health-Related Exercise in the National Curriculum* by Jo Harris, 2001, Champaign, IL: Human Kinetics.

Example: Mapping HRE at Key Stages 1 to 4

The following represents an example of how HRE might be mapped within a school curriculum. For each key stage, the HRE learning outcomes (detailed on pages 36-40) have been placed within the areas of activity or within focused topics or units.

KEY STAGE 1

Activity area	Safety issues	Exercise effects	Health benefits	Activity promotion
Dance	a, b	aiii, aiv, av, b, c	ai	a, b
Games	a, b	ai, aii	ai, aii	a, b
Gymnastics	a, b	avi	aii	a, b
Swimming	—	—	—	—
Topic approach	—	—	—	—

KEY STAGE 2

Activity area	Safety issues	Exercise effects	Health benefits	Activity promotion
Athletics	a, b	ai, aii, aiii	a, c	b, c
Dance	a, b	a	b	b, c
Games	a, b	ai, aii, aiii	b	b, c
Gymnastics	a, b	—	a, c	b, c
OAA	a, b	—	b	b, c
Swimming	a, b	ai, aii	a, c	b, c
Topic approach: My Body	—	a, b	d	a, d

KEY STAGE 3

Activity area	Safety issues	Exercise effects	Health benefits	Activity promotion
Athletics	a, c, d, e	ai, aii, b	d	a, b

Activity area	Safety issues	Exercise effects	Health benefits	Activity promotion
Dance	a, c, d, e	b	d	a, b
Games	a, c, d, e	ai, b	d	a, b
Gymnastics	a, b, c, d, e	aii, b	d	a, b
OAA	a, c, d, e	b	d	a, b
Swimming	a, c, d, e	b	d	a, b
Focused units *Y7: Heart health*	e	ai, b, c	ai-iii, b, c	c, d, e
Y9: Muscle health	c, e	aii, b, c	ai-iii, b, c	d, e
PSHE-PSE	a	—	—	a, b
KEY STAGE 4				
Activity area	**Safety issues**	**Exercise effects**	**Health benefits**	**Activity promotion**
Athletics	a, b	a, b	d	b, di-vii
Dance	a, b	a, b	d	b
Games	a, b	a, b	d	b, di-vii
Gymnastics	a, b	a, b	d	b
OAA	a, b	a, b	d	b
Swimming	a, b, c	a, b	d	b, di-vii
*Sport**	a, b	a, b	d	b, di-vii
*Exercise activities**	c	a, b	d	a, b, c, di-vii
Focused units *Y10: Aerobics, circuits, weight-training*	c	a, b	d	a, b, c, di-vii, e, f
Y11: Personal exercise programme	c	a, b	a, b, c, d	a, b, c, di-vii, e, f
PSHE-PSE	a	—	c	b, e, f

* Applies to the National Curriculum for Physical Education in Wales.

Permeation of HRE Through the Activity Areas

The following table provides examples of a structured, staged approach to delivering some of the HRE learning outcomes through the activity areas.

Safe exercise principles and practices	
Year	**By the end of the year, pupils should achieve the following learning outcomes:**
1	Know and adhere to safety rules and practices such as changing clothes for PE lessons, tying long hair back, removing jewellery
2	Know and adhere to safety rules and practices such as sitting and standing with good posture, wearing footwear when skipping with a rope, no running fast to touch walls
3	Understand the need for safety rules and practices such as adopting good posture at all times, being hygienic
4	Understand the need for safety rules and practices such as changing clothes and washing after energetic activity, wearing footwear for some activities, following rules
5	Understand the need for safety practices such as protecting against cold weather, avoiding sunburn
6	Understand the need for safety practices such as safe lifting, sensible use of space
7	Demonstrate understanding of safe exercise practices (e.g., tying long hair back and removing jewellery to avoid injury; adopting good posture when sitting, standing and moving; performing exercises with good technique; washing or showering following energetic activity; using equipment and facilities with permission and, where necessary, under supervision; administering basic first aid; wearing adequate protection such as goalkeeping gloves and leg pads for certain activities; coping with specific weather conditions such as using sunscreen to avoid burning in hot weather and drinking fluids to prevent dehydration)
8	Demonstrate concern for and understanding of back care by lifting, carrying, placing and using equipment responsibly and with good technique; understand safety procedures associated with specific activities
9	Understand why certain exercises and practices are not recommended (e.g., standing toe touches, straight leg sit-ups, bouncing in stretches, flinging movements) and be able to perform safe alternatives (e.g., seated 'sit and reach', curl-ups with bent legs, holding stretches still, performing movements with control)
10	Be able to recognise risk and apply safe exercise principles and procedures (e.g., not exercising when unwell or injured, avoiding prolonged high-impact exercise)
11	Be able to recognise and manage risk and apply safe exercise principles and procedures (e.g., administering basic first aid, including resuscitation techniques; avoiding excessive amounts of exercise)

Preparation for and recovery from activity	
Year	**By the end of the year, pupils should achieve the following learning outcomes:**
1	Know that activity starts with a gentle warm-up
2	Know that activity finishes with a calming cool-down
3	Know the purpose of a warm-up

Year	By the end of the year, pupils should achieve the following learning outcomes:
4	Recognise and describe parts of a warm-up (i.e., exercise for the joints such as arm circles, whole-body activities such as jogging or skipping without a rope, and stretches for the whole body such as reaching long and tall)
5	Know the purpose of a cool-down
6	Recognise and describe parts of a cool-down (i.e., whole-body activities such as walking, and stretches for the whole body or parts of the body such as the lower leg or calf muscles)
7	Understand the value of preparing for and recovering from activity and the possible consequences of not doing so and be able to explain the purpose of each component of a warm-up and cool-down
8	Be able to plan and perform each component of a warm-up (i.e., mobility exercises, whole-body activities, static stretches) and cool-down (i.e., whole-body activities, static stretches) for general activity (e.g., athletics, dance, games)
9	Be able to plan and perform warm-ups and cool-downs for specific activities (e.g., hockey, high jump, volleyball, circuit-training)
10	Be able to evaluate warm-ups and cool-downs in terms of safety, effectiveness and relevance to the specific activity
11	Take responsibility for their own safe, effective and relevant preparation for and recovery from activity

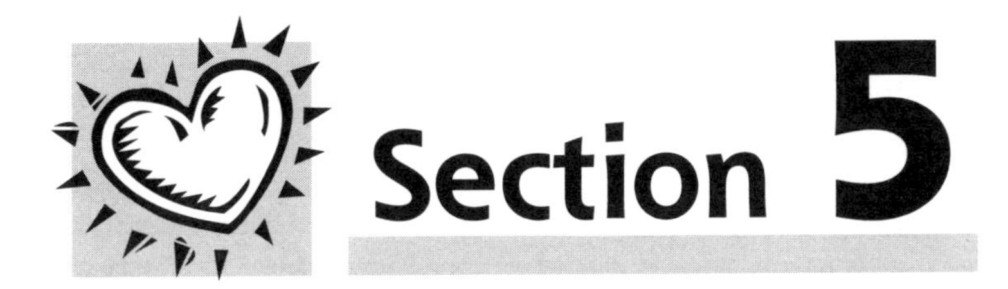

Section 5

Sample Scheme and Units of Work

SAMPLE SCHEME OF WORK FOR HEALTH-RELATED EXERCISE

This section provides a sample scheme of work that meets the health-related exercise (HRE) requirements of the national curriculum for England and for Wales. The scheme is founded on the HRE learning outcomes (pages 36 to 40). Example units of work (pages 52 to 73) support the scheme.

Key Stage 1

During this key stage, pupils focus on exploring how their bodies feel during different activities and understanding how important it is to be active. Pupils learn how to exercise safely and to recognise and describe a range of physical, mental and social effects of exercise. Pupils also learn about good posture, the names of the main external parts of the body, and the source of energy for physical activity. This learning occurs through the programmes of study for dance, games and gymnastics.

Key Stage 2

During this key stage, learning focuses on understanding the short-term effects of exercise, especially those related to the circulatory system. Pupils learn about the physical, mental and social health benefits of exercise, including how physical activity contributes to maintaining a healthy body weight. Pupils continue to be involved in appropriate warm-up and cool-down procedures. They are encouraged to adopt good posture. Pupils become aware of how active they are and should be. They learn about opportunities available to them to be more active in school and in the local community. The programmes of study for the activity areas meet most of the key stage 2 requirements. A topic-based unit 'My Body' (year 6), which combines physical education and science requirements, delivers other concepts.

Key Stage 3

During this key stage, learning focuses on (a) understanding the short- and long-term effects of exercise on the cardiovascular and musculo-skeletal systems and (b) the role that physical activity plays in establishing and maintaining good health, including enhanced social and psychological well-being, and achieving a healthy body weight. Pupils learn how to prepare for, undertake and recover safely and sensibly from specific activities in varying contexts and conditions, and they begin to take responsibility for planning and execution. Pupils learn how to incorporate exercise into their lifestyles and how to become involved in activities that are good for their personal health and well-being. The programmes of study for the activity areas meet some of the key stage 3 requirements. The focused units 'Heart Health' (year 7) and 'Muscle Health' (year 9) deliver other concepts. The school's PSHE programme delivers some health-related issues associated with activity promotion (such as accessing information about activity opportunities in the locality) and basic first aid.

Key Stage 4

During this key stage, learning focuses on designing, carrying out, monitoring, developing and evaluating safe and effective exercise programmes that meet pupils' personal needs and preferences. Pupils take more responsibility for preparing for and recovering from activity, and they learn to apply the key principles of exercise programming and training to selected activities. They learn about the benefits of an active way of life (including the role of exercise in managing stress) and the risks associated with a sedentary lifestyle and with excessive dieting and exercising. Pupils consider constraints to being active and ways they might overcome them to gain access to activity opportunities in the local community. The programmes of study for the selected activities meet some key stage 4 requirements. Focused units on specific fitness activities such as aerobics and circuits (year 10) and follow-up units on step aerobics, weight- training and the unit 'Personal Exercise Programme' (year 11) deliver other concepts. The school's PSHE programme delivers some health-related issues associated with activity and health promotion (such as considering constraints to being active and ways of overcoming them, and the risks associated with excessive dieting and exercising).

INTRODUCTION TO EXAMPLE UNITS OF WORK

Sample units of work are presented for each of the four key stages. The samples cover a range of approaches to the delivery of HRE including permeation through the activity areas, focused units and a topic-based approach. Each unit includes the following sections:

Objectives: a statement of what the pupils will be taught
National curriculum links: links with relevant aspects of the National Curriculum for Physical Education and related subjects

Learning outcomes: a description of what a pupil should know, understand and be able to do as a result of taking part in the lessons

Learning activities: an indication of what the pupils will do in lessons to realise the learning outcomes

Assessment: identification of when assessment opportunities might arise as pupils engage in activities (the numbers refer to the planned learning outcomes)

Resources: the requirements for teaching the unit

The units provide examples of the delivery of HRE through the areas of activity. Examples of permeated learning outcomes are listed here. Pupils should be able to do the following:

- » Recognise and describe how their bodies feel when playing invasion games
- » Sit and stand with good posture and know that activity starts with a gentle warm-up and finishes with a calming cool-down
- » Name parts of the body, recognise and describe how their muscles feel when taking part in jumps, rolls and balances, and know that regular exercise helps body parts to grow, develop and work well
- » Understand about hygiene and recognise and describe parts of a warm-up
- » Understand how traditional dancing affects the body in the short term and why dancing is good for their health and well-being
- » Understand the need to protect the body in certain weather and know the purpose of a cool-down
- » Demonstrate understanding of safe exercise practice and back care and the value and purpose of each component of a warm-up and cool-down
- » Understand the short-term effects and long-term benefits of weight-bearing gymnastic activities
- » Understand the effects and benefits of running
- » Plan and perform safe and effective warm-ups and cool-downs for running activities
- » Demonstrate understanding of safe exercise practice and plan and perform warm-up and cool-down routines relevant to the game of hockey
- » Plan, perform, monitor and evaluate effective personal training programmes for their selected events, showing understanding of the principles involved

The examples also show how focused units might deliver aspects of HRE. Examples of learning outcomes delivered in this way are listed here. Pupils should be able to do the following:

- » Understand the effect of exercise and rest on pulse rate and the short-term effects and health benefits of exercise
- » Understand the short-term effects and long-term benefits of cardiovascular exercise on health, fitness and performance
- » Compare their activity levels with the exercise recommendations for young people
- » Understand the role of activity in healthy weight management
- » Perform with good technique a range of strength and flexibility exercises associated with good posture
- » Understand the short-term effects and long-term benefits of musculo-skeletal exercise on health, fitness and performance
- » Understand why certain strength and flexibility exercises are not recommended and be able to perform safe alternatives
- » Perform with good technique a range of safe, effective aerobics steps and actions
- » Plan, perform and evaluate the components of an aerobics class
- » Understand and apply the principles associated with designing, carrying out, monitoring and developing a safe, effective aerobics workout
- » Understand the short-term effects and long-term benefits of weight-training and factors affecting participation
- » Take responsibility for their own safe, effective and relevant preparation for and recovery from weight-training

>> Plan, perform, monitor and evaluate a safe, effective health-related exercise programme that meets their personal needs and preferences over an extended period

Example Unit: Delivering HRE Through Games at Key Stage 1

Invasion games	**National curriculum links**	
YEAR 1 **Objectives** This unit should enable pupils to do the following: • Travel with, send and receive a ball in different ways • Develop these skills and play simple invasion-type games • Know and adhere to safety practices for games (e.g., wearing suitable PE kit for games, tying long hair back, removing jewellery) and know that activity starts with a gentle warm-up • Recognise and describe how their bodies feel when playing invasion games (focusing on breathing and heart rate)	**ENGLAND** **Games programme of study** Pupils should be taught to travel with, send and receive a ball in different ways; develop these skills for simple invasion-type games; and play simple invasion-type games. **Knowledge and understanding of fitness and health** Pupils should be taught to recognise and describe how their bodies feel during different activities.	**WALES** **Games programme of study** Pupils should be taught to use elements of play that promote spatial awareness, which include running, chasing and dodging to avoid others; to create and develop simple co-operative and competitive games and to play these fairly and safely, first individually and, when ready, in pairs and small groups; and to develop and practise a variety of ways of sending, receiving and travelling with a ball. **Health-related exercise** Pupils should be taught about the changes that happen to their bodies as they exercise, how to recognise the effects, and how to describe changes to their breathing and heart rate.

Learning outcomes (LOs)	**Learning activities**	**Assessment of LOs**	**Resources**
Pupils should be able to do the following:	This unit should provide opportunities for pupils to do the following:		
1. Adhere to safety practices and follow relevant warm-up activities	Be informed about safety practices relevant to games and engage in simple games-related activities such as moving safely in open and confined spaces	1	Cones, line markings
2. Roll, kick and travel with a ball in a controlled manner	Send a ball by rolling it to a partner	2	Balls, cones, line markings
	Send a ball by kicking it to a partner	2	
	Travel around a partner or cone carrying or kicking a ball	2	
3. Receive a ball that has been rolled or kicked to them while they are stationary	Receive a ball that has been rolled or kicked	3	
4. Play simple invasion-type games	Play simple games in pairs and small groups that incorporate rolling or kicking, receiving, travelling with the ball and running and chasing (e.g., how many passes in 30 seconds? how many people can you tag in 60 seconds?)	4	Balls, cones, line markings, bibs or bands
5. Recognise and describe the effects of playing invasion games on their breathing and heart rate	Experience and describe how playing invasion games makes their hearts pump more quickly and makes them breathe faster and deeper	5	Breathing and heart rate charts (e.g., a scale ranging from very slow to very fast)

Example Unit: Delivering HRE Through Gymnastics at Key Stage 1

Gymnastics	National curriculum links	
YEAR 2 **Objectives** This unit should enable pupils to do the following: • Develop the range of their jumping, rolling and balancing actions • Select and link jumping, rolling and balancing actions in short movement phrases • Sit and stand with good posture and know that activity starts with a gentle warm-up and finishes with a calming cool-down • Name parts of the body, recognise and describe how their muscles feel when taking part in jumps, rolls and balances, and know that regular exercise helps body parts grow, develop and work well	**ENGLAND** **Gymnastics programme of study** Pupils should be taught to perform basic skills in travelling, being still, finding space and using it safely, both on the floor and using apparatus; to develop the range of their skills and actions; to choose and link skills and actions in short movement phrases; and to create and perform short, linked sequences that show a clear beginning, middle and end and have contrasts in direction, level and speed. **Knowledge and understanding of fitness and health** Pupils should be taught how important it is to be active and to recognise and describe how their bodies feel during different activities. **Science programme of study** Pupils should be taught to recognise and compare the main external parts of the bodies of humans and other animals. **PSHE and citizenship** Pupils should be taught the names of the main parts of the body.	**WALES** **Gymnastics programme of study** Pupils should be taught to use the basic actions of travelling including jumping and landing, transferring weight from feet to hands, balancing, rolling, both on the floor and when using apparatus; to develop the basic actions in sequences, improving their control and use of different shapes, levels and direction of travel; and to lift, carry, place and use apparatus safely. **Health-related exercise** Pupils should be taught to understand the changes that happen to their bodies as they exercise; to recognise the effects and describe changes; to adopt good posture when sitting, standing and taking part in activity; to prepare for and recover from activity appropriately; and to realise that exercise helps body parts work well. **Science programme of study** Pupils should be taught to name the main external parts of the human body and to understand that exercising helps humans to keep healthy. **Personal and social education** Pupils should value being healthy, be positive about the actions necessary to be healthy, and know that exercise is important to keep their bodies healthy.

Learning outcomes (LOs)	Learning activities	Assessment of LOs	Resources
Pupils should be able to do the following: 1. Gently prepare for and calmly recover from gymnastic activity and know what is meant by good posture 2. Perform a variety of jumps, rolls and balances and select suitable actions to	This unit should provide opportunities for pupils to do the following:		
	Sit and stand with good posture and travel on their feet in different ways, holding a still position (such as a balance or stretch) on command	1	Appropriate distribution of mats
	Explore and practise jumps showing different shapes in the air	2	Appropriate distribution of mats
	Explore and practise rolls showing different shapes	2	Appropriate distribution of mats

(continued)

Example Unit: Delivering HRE Through Gymnastics at Key Stage 1 *(continued)*

Learning outcomes (LOs)	Learning activities	Assessment of LOs	Resources
include in a sequence	Explore and practise balances altering the size and number of the base points	2	
3. Recognise and describe how muscles feel during 'still' and 'moving' gymnastic actions and know the benefits of such actions	Name major body parts (e.g., hands, feet, bones, muscles), recognise and describe how their muscles feel both when moving (e.g., jump or roll) and holding a body shape (e.g., balance), and appreciate that regular exercise helps bones and muscles grow, develop and work well	3	Visual aid of muscles and skeleton
	Select their best jumps, rolls and balances and put them together to form a short sequence	2, 4	Appropriate distribution of mats
4. Perform and link a series of jumps, rolls and balances on the floor and on low apparatus	On low apparatus, link together a series of different jumps, rolls and balances	4	Appropriate apparatus (e.g., benches, low box-tops, low balancing tables, mats)

Example Unit: Delivering HRE Through Dance at Key Stage 2

Traditional dancing	National curriculum links	
YEAR 4 **Objectives** This unit should enable pupils to do the following: • Perform and develop an appreciation of traditional dances from different times and places • Compose their own dances using simple movement patterns from traditional dances from different times and places • Understand about hygiene (e.g., the need to change clothing and wash after energetic activity) and recognise and describe parts of a warm-up • Understand how traditional dancing affects the body in the short term (breathing rate, heart rate, body temperature, feelings) and why dancing is good for their health and well-being	**ENGLAND** **Dance programme of study** Pupils should be taught to create and perform dances using a range of movement patterns, including those from different times, places and cultures. **Knowledge and understanding of fitness and health** Pupils should be taught how exercise affects the body in the short term, how to warm up and prepare appropriately for different activities, why physical activity is good for their health and well-being, and why wearing appropriate clothing and being hygienic is good for their health and safety.	**WALES** **Dance programme of study** Pupils should be taught to compose, perform and appreciate phrases, motifs and whole dances with increased control, sensitivity, sense of rhythm and clarity of body shape. Pupils should be given opportunities to perform and develop an appreciation of dances from different traditions, times and places, including some traditional dances from Wales. **Health-related exercise** Pupils should be taught to sustain activity over appropriate periods in a range of physical activities; to understand the short-term effects of exercise on the body; to adopt good posture when sitting, standing and taking part in activity; to prepare for and recover from activity appropriately; and to recognise that exercise can be fun and sociable.

Learning outcomes (LOs)	Learning activities	Assessment of LOs	Resources
Pupils should be able to do the following:	This unit should provide opportunities for pupils to do the following:		
1. Understand about hygiene and recognise and describe parts of a warm-up 2. Perform a range of traditional dances with control 3. Compose, perform and appreciate traditional dance movement pattens 4. Explain the effects of performing traditional dances on breathing rate, heart rate, body temperature and feelings	Be informed and follow guidance about good hygiene (e.g., changing clothes and washing after energetic activity)	1	
	Recognise and describe different parts of a warm-up (e.g., joint actions such as shoulder circles and knee bends, whole-body activities such as walking, skipping and galloping to warm the body, and whole-body stretches such as reaching long and tall or far and wide to prepare the muscles)	1	
	Familiarise themselves with the rhythm of the music using body actions (e.g., clapping, foot tapping, skipping) and by practising a range of movement patterns in time with the music	2	Music machine, tapes or CDs, instructions
	Perform a range of movement patterns from traditional dances (e.g., galloping, 'do-si-dos', circles, right- and left-hand stars) and describe the patterns in terms of (i) actions (e.g., clap, gallop, skip, walk), (ii) directions (e.g., forward, backwards, sideways), and (iii) shapes (e.g., circles, lines, stars)	2	Music machine, tapes or CDs, posters to summarise actions, directions and shapes
	Compose their own movement patterns combining actions, directions or shapes (e.g., skipping forwards in a circle)	3	Music machine, tapes or CDs
	Monitor their breathing, heart rate and body temperature (e.g., feel their foreheads, chests and over their mouths) before and after a sustained period of energetic dancing and offer simple explanations for the effects (e.g, my heart is beating faster to get more blood to the muscles in the arms and legs)	4	Charts (e.g., scales ranging from 'very fast or hot' to 'very slow or cold')
	Appreciate that dancing can be enjoyable, fun and sociable	4	

Example Unit: Delivering HRE Through Net Games at Key Stage 2

Short tennis	National curriculum links	
YEAR 5 **Objectives** This unit should enable pupils to do the following: • Improve the skills of sending, receiving and striking a ball in preparation for playing small-sided, modified net games	**ENGLAND** **Games programme of study** Pupils should be taught to play and make up small-sided and modified competitive net games, use skills and tactics and apply basic principles suitable for attacking and defending, and work with others to organise and keep games going.	**WALES** **Games programme of study** Pupils should be taught to play small-sided, modified versions of net games, focusing on common skills and principles, including attack and defence; to develop the skills of sending, receiving and striking a ball; and to understand

(continued)

Example Unit: Delivering HRE Through Net Games at Key Stage 2 *(continued)*

Short tennis	**National curriculum links**	
YEAR 5	**ENGLAND**	**WALES**
• Apply basic principles of attack and defence in net games • Understand the need to protect the body in certain weather conditions and know the purpose of a cool-down • Understand the effects on the body of playing net games	**Knowledge and understanding of fitness and health** Pupils should be taught how exercise affects the body in the short term, how to warm up and prepare appropriately for different activities, why physical activity is good for their health and well-being, and why wearing appropriate clothing and being hygienic is good for their health and safety.	the structure of games, including their rules and scoring systems. Pupils should have opportunities to observe the conventions of fair play, honest competition and good sporting behaviour as individual participants and team members. **Health-related exercise** Pupils should be taught to sustain activity over appropriate periods in a range of physical activities; to understand the short-term effects of exercise on the body; to adopt good posture when sitting, standing and taking part in activity; to prepare for and recover from activity appropriately; to understand that exercise strengthens bones and muscles; to recognise that exercise can be fun and sociable; and to know that exercise should be done every day for it to be beneficial.

Learning outcomes (LOs)	**Learning activities**	**Assessment of LOs**	**Resources**
Pupils should be able to do the following: 1. Understand the need to protect the body in cold and hot weather and know the purpose of a cool-down 2. Send, receive and strike a ball with control and accuracy 3. Understand the basic principles of attack and defence in net games 4. Understand the changes that happen to their bodies during net games	This unit should provide opportunities for pupils to do the following:		
	Explain the need to protect the body in cold and hot weather (e.g., covering exposed parts of the body to avoid burning or getting very cold)	1	
	Explain the purpose of a cool-down (i.e., to recover comfortably from energetic activity by gradually slowing down and calming the body)	1	Cones, line markings
	Throw and catch a ball over different distances and at varying speeds	2	Balls and rackets (of varying size, shape and weight), markers
	Strike a stationary and moving ball with control and in a given direction	2	
	Describe basic principles of attacking play in net games (e.g., playing the ball into open space away from the opponent)	3	Balls, rackets, net or wall boundary (of an appropriate height)
	Describe basic principles of defending play in net games (e.g., being ready to cover the space and return a ball on either side of the body)	3	Balls, rackets, net or wall boundary (of an appropriate height)
	Explain the physical, mental and social effects of playing net games (e.g., changes in breathing rate, heart rate, body temperature, appearance; stronger heart, lungs, bones and muscles; fun, enjoyment, cooperation)	4	Posters, worksheets

Example Unit: Delivering HRE Within a Topic Approach at Key Stage 2

<table>
<tr><th>Topic 'My Body'
(physical education and science)</th><th colspan="2">National curriculum links</th></tr>
<tr><td>YEAR 6

Objectives

This unit should enable pupils to do the following:
• Understand that the heart works as a pump to circulate blood around the body
• Understand the effect of exercise and rest on pulse rate and the short-term effects and health benefits of exercise
• Understand the effect of food, drink and activity on body weight
• Be aware of their current levels of activity and the need to be active every day</td><td>ENGLAND

Knowledge and understanding of fitness and health

Pupils should be taught how exercise affects the body in the short term, how to warm up and prepare appropriately for different activities, why physical activity is good for their health and well-being, and why wearing appropriate clothing and being hygienic is good for their health and safety.

Science programme of study

Pupils should be taught about the need for food for activity and growth and about the importance of an adequate and varied diet for health; that the heart works as a pump to circulate the blood through vessels around the body, including through the lungs; about the effect of exercise and rest on pulse rate; and about the importance of exercise for good health.

PSHE and citizenship

Pupils should be taught what makes a healthy lifestyle, including the benefits of exercise and healthy eating; what affects mental health; and how to make informed choices.</td><td>WALES

Health-related exercise

Pupils should be taught to sustain activity over appropriate periods in a range of physical activities; to understand the short-term effects of exercise on the body; to recognise that the body needs a certain amount of energy for activity and that if more food and drink is taken in than is needed for activity then body fat increases; to understand that exercise strengthens bones and muscles; to recognise that exercise can be fun and sociable; and to know exercise should be done every day for it to be beneficial.

Science programme of study

Pupils should be taught that the body needs different foods for activity and growth, that an adequate and varied diet is needed to keep healthy, that the heart acts as a pump, that blood circulates in the body through arteries and veins, that the pulse gives a measure of the heart beat rate, and that exercise and rest affect pulse rate.

Personal and social education

Pupils should understand the benefits of exercise and hygiene and the need for a variety of food for growth and activity.</td></tr>
</table>

<table>
<tr><th>Learning outcomes (LOs)</th><th>Learning activities</th><th>Assessment of LOs</th><th>Resources</th></tr>
<tr><td rowspan="3">Pupils should be able to do the following:
1. Demonstrate knowledge of the circulatory system and of the heart's structure and function
2. Understand the effect of exercise on the pulse rate and the short-term</td><td>This unit should provide opportunities for pupils to do the following:</td><td></td><td></td></tr>
<tr><td>Locate and recognise the different parts of the circulatory system (heart, lungs, blood vessels) and find out about and discuss their functions (classroom)</td><td>1</td><td>Diagrams, posters, books, CD-ROMs, model</td></tr>
<tr><td>Explore how oxygen travels in the blood during a physical education lesson (e.g., 'circulatory circuit' involving continuous travel from the 'muscles' to the 'lungs', back through the 'heart' and to the 'muscles' again; the circuit can be walked and then jogged and different actions can be</td><td>1</td><td>Equipment for selected activity (e.g., cones, task cards, posters)</td></tr>
</table>

(continued)

Example Unit: Delivering HRE Within a Topic Approach at Key Stage 2 *(continued)*

Learning outcomes (LOs)	Learning activities	Assessment of LOs	Resources
effects of exercise on the body 3. Understand the effect of food, drink and activity on body weight 4. Become aware of their current activity level and of opportunities to be active every day	performed at various parts of the system such as energetic jumping in the 'muscles' and taking deep breaths in the 'lungs')		
	Measure and record their pulse rates and breathing rates before and after energetic activity during a physical eduation lesson (e.g., skipping activities) and explain the differences	2	Equipment for selected activity (e.g., skipping ropes)
	Understand that the body needs a certain amount of energy every day in food and drink to function properly, that body fat increases if more food and drink are taken in than is needed, and that being active helps to maintain a healthy body weight	3	Diagrams, posters, model
	Discuss their current levels of activity (e.g., daily, twice a week) and consider opportunities to be active on a daily basis (e.g., walking or cycling to school, playing sport) (classroom)	4	Simple activity questionnaire or diary, charts, posters

Example Unit: Delivering HRE Through Gymnastics at Key Stage 3

Gymnastics	National curriculum links	
YEAR 7 **Objectives** This unit should enable pupils to do the following: • Refine travelling, twisting and turning actions and improve the quality of performance through increased tension and extension • Create and perform individual and partner sequences on the floor and apparatus showing contrasts in speed, direction and level • Demonstrate their understanding of safe exercise practice and back care and the value and purpose of each component of a warm-up and cool-down • Understand the short-term effects and long-term benefits of weight-bearing gymnastic activities	**ENGLAND** **Gymnastics programme of study** Pupils should be taught to create and perform complex sequences on the floor and using apparatus, use techniques and movement combinations in different gymnastic styles, and use compositional principles when designing their sequences. **Knowledge and understanding of fitness and health** Pupils should be taught how to prepare for and recover from specific activities, how different types of activity affect specific aspects of their fitness, how they will benefit from regular exercise and good hygiene, and how to become involved in activities that are good for their personal and social health and well-being.	**WALES** **Gymnastics programme of study** Pupils should be taught to adapt, refine and increase their range of gymnastic actions on the floor and apparatus, alone or with others, involving travelling, twisting and turning; to refine a series of gymnastic actions into increasingly complex sequences using both the floor and apparatus that show variety, contrast and repetition; to understand the factors that promote quality in gymnastic performances, including body tension and extension; and to lift, carry, place and use apparatus safely. **Health-related exercise** Pupils should be taught to monitor a range of short-term effects on the musculo-skeletal system; to appreciate the long-term effects of exercise on physical health; to adopt good posture when sitting, standing and taking part in activity; to use relevant and safe warm-up and cool-down routines and to take responsibility for their planning

Gymnastics	National curriculum links	
		and execution; to realise that appropriate training can improve fitness and performance; and to know the value of exercise to social and psychological well-being.

Learning outcomes (LOs)	Learning activities	Assessment of LOs	Resources
Pupils should be able to do the following:	This unit should provide opportunities for pupils to do the following:		
1. Perform a range of travelling, twisting and turning actions both on the floor and using small and large apparatus 2. Plan, perform and evaluate sequences alone and with a partner showing contrasts in speed, direction and level 3. Demonstrate and explain how body tension helps to improve the quality of gymnastic actions 4. Demonstrate an understanding of safe exercise practice, back care and the value and purpose of parts of a warm-up and cool-down 5. Explain the short-term effects and long-term benefits of gymnastic actions	Explain safe exercise practices (e.g., removing jewellery to avoid injury, adopting good posture, using equipment with permission) and demonstrate their concern for and understanding of back care by lifting, carrying, placing and using equipment responsibly and with good technique	4	Posters, charts
	Explain the value of safely and effectively preparing for and recovering from gymnastics and the consequences of not doing so (discomfort, injury) and the purpose of each component of a warm-up and cool-down (mobility exercises, whole-body activities, static stretches)	4	Task cards, prompt sheets
	Practise and refine a variety of travelling, twisting and turning actions with contrasts in speed (e.g., fast bursts followed by sustained activity), direction (e.g., forward, backward, diagonal) and level (e.g., high, medium, low) both on the floor and using small and large apparatus, and demonstrate how to show body tension and extension during such actions (e.g., by pointing toes and pulling in abdominal muscles)	1,3	Mats, small and large apparatus
	Explore how partners can work in contrast to each other in speed, direction and level; plan, perform and evaluate sequences alone and with a partner that combine travelling, twisting and turning actions; and show contrasts in speed, direction and level, and body tension and extension	2,3	Mats, small and large apparatus, task cards, digital camera, video
	Describe what is happening to their bodies in gymnastics (i.e., muscles pull on bones to lift, lower and control) and explain the short-term effects (i.e., increased muscular strength, endurance and flexibility; improved muscle tone and posture; strengthened bones; enhanced functional capacity, sport performance, sense of achievement) and long-term benefits of gymnastic activities (assists weight management, reduces risk of osteoporosis and back pain, improves management of arthritis)	5	Charts, posters, CD-ROMs, visual aids

Example Focused Unit: Delivering HRE at Key Stage 3

Heart health	National curriculum links	
YEAR 7 **Objectives** This unit should enable pupils to do the following: • Perform a range of safe and effective cardiovascular activities with good technique and monitor a range of their short-term effects • Understand the short-term effects and long-term benefits of cardiovascular exercise on health, fitness and performance • Compare their activity levels with the exercise recommendations for young people • Understand the role of activity in healthy weight management	**ENGLAND** **Knowledge and understanding of fitness and health** Pupils should be taught how different types of activity affect specific aspects of their fitness, how they will benefit from regular exercise and good hygiene, and how to become involved in activities that are good for their personal and social health and well-being. **Science programme of study** Pupils should be taught about the need for a balanced diet containing carbohydrates, proteins, fats, minerals, vitamins, fibre and water, and about the foods that are sources of these; that food is used as a fuel during respiration to maintain the body's activity and as a raw material for growth and repair; and that aerobic respiration involves a reaction in cells between oxygen and food in which glucose is broken down into carbon dioxide and water.	**WALES** **Health-related exercise** Pupils should be taught to monitor a range of short-term effects on the cardiovascular system; to appreciate the long-term effects of exercise on physical health; to know the differences between whole-body activities that help to reduce body fat and conditioning exercises that improve muscle tone; to realise that appropriate training can improve fitness and performance; to know the value of exercise to social and psychological well-being; and to become aware of the range of activity opportunities at school, home and in the local community, and ways of incorporating exercise into their lifestyles. **Science programme of study** Pupils should be taught that food is used as a fuel during respiration to maintain the body's activity and as a raw material for growth and repair; that aerobic respiration is a reaction in cells in which glucose reacts with oxygen and is broken down into carbon dioxide and water; and that aerobic respiration provides energy for use by the body.

Learning outcomes (LOs)	Learning activities	Assessment of LOs	Resources
Pupils should be able to do the following: 1. Perform a range of cardiovascular activities with good technique 2. Monitor and understand the short-term effects of cardiovascular exercise 3. Understand the long-term benefits of cardiovascular exercise	This unit should provide opportunities for pupils to do the following: Perform a range of cardiovascular activities (e.g., brisk walking, jogging, running, skipping, active games playing, swimming, exercising to music) with good technique and understand the consequences of poor technique (e.g., jogging or skipping on toes; performing uncontrolled, flinging movements)	1	As appropriate for the activities (e.g., skipping ropes), digital camera, video
	Monitor and explain the range of short-term effects of cardiovascular exercise (e.g., changes in breathing and heart rate, recovery rate, temperature, appearance, feelings) and be aware of what 'moderate intensity' and 'vigorous intensity' exercise feel like (e.g., working within a range of moderate to vigorous exercise)	2	Equipment (e.g., watch, tapes, sportstesters, graphic calculator), worksheets, exertion scales (e.g., 'very easy' to 'very hard' gears)

Learning outcomes (LOs)	Learning activities	Assessment of LOs	Resources
4. Compare their activity levels with those recommended for young people 5. Understand the role of exercise in healthy weight management	Explain the range of long-term benefits of cardiovascular exercise on physical health (e.g., reduced risk of heart disease, obesity) on mental and social health (e.g., enjoying being with friends, increased confidence and self-esteem, decreased anxiety and stress) and on fitness and performance (both enhanced), and appreciate that an appropriate balance among work, leisure and exercise promotes good health	3	Posters, charts, worksheets
	Develop their awareness of the exercise recommendations for young people (60 minutes of at least moderate-intensity activity per day, 30 minutes for the currently inactive), monitor their activity levels (using diaries over four to six weeks) and compare them with the recommendations for young people	4	Posters, charts, worksheets, activity diaries
	Explain the energy balance equation involving energy intake (food and drink) and energy expenditure (activity) and how this relates to maintaining a healthy body weight (e.g., cardiovascular activities use large muscles in the whole body, expending energy and helping to reduce body fat), know that the body needs a minimum daily energy intake to function properly, and know that strict dieting and excessive exercising can damage one's health	5	Posters, charts (e.g., energy balance equation)

Example Unit: Delivering HRE Through Cross-Country Running at Key Stage 3

Cross-country running	National curriculum links	
YEAR 8 **Objectives** This unit should enable pupils to do the following: • Perform with good technique a range of running activities and challenges • Understand the effects and benefits of running • Plan and perform safe and effective warm-ups and cool-downs for running activities	**ENGLAND** **Athletics programme of study** Pupils should be taught to set and meet personal and group targets in a range of athletic events, challenges and competitions and use a range of running techniques, singly and in combination, with precision, speed, power or stamina. **Knowledge and understanding of fitness and health** Pupils should be taught how to prepare for and recover from specific activities, how different types of activity affect specific aspects of their fitness, how they will benefit from regular exercise and good hygiene,	**WALES** **Athletics programme of study** Pupils should be taught to apply the techniques, skills and competition rules specific to at least one running event, to apply the relevant mechanical principles underpinning performance in selected events, and to understand the effects of taking part in a sustained event compared with an event of a more explosive nature. Pupils should be given opportunities to improve performance through setting targets to beat previous best performance. **Health-related exercise** Pupils should be taught to monitor a range of short-term effects on the

(continued)

Cross-country running	**National curriculum links**	
YEAR 8	**ENGLAND**	**WALES**
	and how to become involved in activities that are good for their personal and social health and well-being.	cardiovascular system; to appreciate the long-term effects of exercise on physical health; to adopt good posture when sitting, standing and taking part in activity; to use relevant and safe warm-up and cool-down routines and take responsibility for their planning and execution; to understand the differences between whole-body activities that help reduce body fat and conditioning exercises that improve muscle tone; to realise that appropriate training can improve fitness and performance; to know the value of exercise to social and psychological well-being; and to become aware of the range of activity opportunities at school, home and in the local community, and ways of incorporating exercise into their lifestyles.

Learning outcomes (LOs)	**Learning activities**	**Assessment of LOs**	**Resources**
Pupils should be able to do the following: 1. Perform a range of running activities and challenges with safe, effective technique 2. Plan and perform warm-ups and cool-downs relevant to running 3. Understand the short-term effects and long-term benefits of running 4. Explain the safety procedures associated with participation in running activities and know where they can participate in the community	This unit should provide opportunities for pupils to do the following:		
	Perform and practise a range of running activities (e.g., jogging, hill-running, fartlek) and challenges, for example, (i) orienteering, timed scavenger hunts, trail chases or pursuits, 'Murder Mystery' event; (ii) whole-group or team challenges (e.g., running the mileage involved in a return trip to London, completing a route in a time calculated by the team); or (iii) personalised challenges (e.g., setting targets to beat previous best time or distance)	1	Cones, markers, flags, watches, bibs or bands
	Describe good running technique (e.g., knee alignment, heel strike, relaxed shoulders), evaluate their own and others' technique and explain safety procedures (e.g., wear visible or reflective clothing and supportive, well-cushioned footwear; tell someone of route and expected time of return; jog with others)	4	Task cards, prompt sheets
	Perform safe, effective warm-ups and cool-downs relevant for running; explain the purpose of the components of a warm-up (mobility exercises, whole-body activities and static stretches) and cool-down (whole-body activities and static stretches); and plan and perform their running	2	Cones, markers, flags, watches, bibs or bands

Learning outcomes (LOs)	Learning activities	Assessment of LOs	Resources
	warm-ups and cool-downs (which should include stretches for the calf and quad muscles)		
	Gradually build up a personal time over which they can sustain steady-paced running	1	Record sheets, watches, sportstester, pedometer
	Monitor and explain the effects of running (e.g., improvements in recovery rate, ability to pace oneself and remain within a target zone) and the benefits (e.g., improved cardiovascular fitness, functional capacity and sport performance; reduced risk of heart disease, osteoporosis, obesity; improved management of asthma; increased opportunities to meet others; decreased anxiety, stress)	3	Posters, charts, CD-ROMs, videos
	Explore and discuss where they can take part in jogging or running (e.g., local running or athletics club, at home, at school)	4	Noticeboards, posters, leaflets, brochures

Example Unit: Delivering HRE Through Invasion Games at Key Stage 3

Hockey

YEAR 9

Objectives

This unit should enable pupils to do the following:

- Refine passing and shooting skills, develop marking and dodging skills and know how to support team members in attack and defense
- Develop knowledge of and perform contrasting team positions
- Demonstrate understanding of safe exercise practice and plan and perform warm-up and cool-down routines relevant to the game of hockey

National curriculum links

ENGLAND

Games programme of study

Pupils should be taught to play competitive invasion games using techniques that suit the games, use the principles of attack and defence when planning and implementing complex team strategies, and respond to changing situations in games.

Knowledge and understanding of fitness and health

Pupils should be taught how to prepare for and recover from specific activities, how different types of activity affect specific aspects of their fitness, how they will benefit from regular exercise and good hygiene, and how to become involved in activities that are good for their personal and social health and well-being.

WALES

Games programme of study

Pupils should be taught a variety of team games, working from small-sided and modified versions to the recognised form, including an invasion game; the techniques, skills, strategies and tactics applicable to selected, recognised games; and the rules, laws and scoring systems specific to selected games. Pupils should be given opportunities to observe the conventions of fair play, honest competition and good sporting behaviour as individual participants and team members.

Health-related exercise

Pupils should be taught to monitor a range of short-term effects on the cardiovascular system; to appreciate the long-term effects of exercise on physical health; to adopt good posture when sitting, standing and taking part in activity; to use relevant and safe

(continued)

Hockey	**National curriculum links**	
YEAR 8	**ENGLAND**	**WALES** warm-up and cool-down routines and to take responsibility for their planning and execution; to realise that appropriate training can improve fitness and performance; to know the value of exercise to social and psychological well-being; and to become aware of the range of activity opportunities at school, home and in the local community and ways of incorporating exercise into their lifestyles.

Learning outcomes (LOs)	**Learning activities**	**Assessment of LOs**	**Resources**
Pupils should be able to do the following: 1. Refine passing and shooting skills and develop marking and dodging skills, including how and when to provide support to team members in attack and defence 2. Play two contrasting team positions (e.g., defender and attacker), showing an understanding of relevant rules and roles in attack and defence 3. Demonstrate understanding of safe exercise practice and plan and perform an appropriate warm-up and cool-down for hockey	This unit should provide opportunities for pupils to do the following:		
	Explain safe exercise practices (e.g., tying long hair back and removing jewellery to avoid injury; wearing adequate protection such as hockey boots, shin pads and goalkeeping gloves and pads)	3	Protective equipment (e.g., goalkeeping gloves and leg pads)
	Experience, understand and then plan and perform safe and effective warm-up and cool-down activities that mobilise joints, warm the body and stretch muscles relevant to the game of hockey (i.e., involve actions, skills, joints and muscles used when playing hockey)	3	Equipment appropriate for the activities (e.g., balls, hockey sticks, cones)
	Practise and refine accurate passing and shooting skills, varying distance and speed and showing awareness of others' strengths and limitations	1	Ball among two or three players
	Develop and practise marking and dodging skills in small-sided modified games (e.g., 3v1; 3v2, 4v3, 4v4, 5v5) and be involved in decision-making both in attack (e.g., how and when to pass, dodge, shoot) and in defense (e.g., how and when to tackle, intercept)	1	Balls, goals, cones, bibs or bands; task cards
	Select two contrasting positions to develop over time within a game (e.g., goalkeeper, right wing), know the role requirements both in attack and in defence, refine the skills required by the particular roles selected (e.g., passing, shooting, kicking, marking, dodging skills) and know the rules of hockey particularly as they apply to those positions	2	Balls, goals, cones, bibs or bands

Example Focused Unit: Delivering HRE at Key Stage 3

Muscle health	National curriculum links	
YEAR 9 **Objectives** This unit should enable pupils to do the following: • Perform with good technique a range of strength and flexibility exercises associated with good posture and monitor a range of short-term effects • Understand the short-term effects and long-term benefits of musculo-skeletal exercise on health, fitness and performance • Understand why certain strength and flexibility exercises are not recommended and be able to perform safe alternatives • Know the exercise recommendations for young people and be aware of activity opportunities in the community	**ENGLAND** **Knowledge and understanding of fitness and health** Pupils should be taught how different types of activity affect specific aspects of their fitness, how they will benefit from regular exercise and good hygiene, and how to become involved in activities that are good for their personal and social health and well-being. **Science programme of study** Pupils should be taught the role of the skeleton and joints and the principle of antagonistic muscle pairs (e.g., biceps and triceps) in movement.	**WALES** **Health-related exercise** Pupils should be taught to monitor a range of short-term effects on the musculo-skeletal system; to appreciate the long-term effects of exercise on physical health; to adopt good posture when sitting, standing and taking part in activity; to understand the differences between whole-body activities that help to reduce body fat and conditioning exercises that improve muscle tone; to realise that appropriate training can improve fitness and performance; to know the value of exercise to social and psychological well-being; and to become aware of the range of activity opportunities at school, home and in the local community and ways of incorporating exercise into their lifestyles. **Science programme of study** Pupils should be taught the role of the skeleton, joints and muscles in movement and the principle of antagonistic muscle pairs (e.g., biceps and triceps).

Learning outcomes (LOs)	Learning activities	Assessment of LOs	Resources
Pupils should be able to do the following:	This unit should provide opportunities for pupils to do the following:		
1. Perform safe, effective and developmentally appropriate strength and flexibility exercises with good technique for the major muscle groups associated with good posture 2. Know the location and names of the major muscle groups associated with good posture	Experience how muscles feel when they are contracting (e.g., firm, hard, warm) or being stretched (e.g., lengthened with mild tension) and identify which muscles need to be (i) strong to support the spine (i.e., the straight and diagonal abdominal muscles, the back muscles, the buttock muscles) and (ii) flexible to maintain correct alignment of the spine (i.e., the hamstrings, hip flexors, chest muscles)	2, 3	Muscle and skeleton posters, visual aids (e.g., muscle model), CD-ROMs
	Select appropriate versions (i.e., easy, moderate, difficult) of and perform with good technique exercises for the major postural muscles—(i) strength exercises (curl-ups, back raises, twisting curl-ups, rear leg lifts, shoulder squeezes) and (ii) stretches (hamstrings, lower back, hip flexors, chest)—and understand why	1	Differentiated circuit cards, mats, light resistance equipment (e.g., bands or elastics, hand weights), music machine, tapes or CDs

(continued)

Learning outcomes (LOs)	Learning activities	Assessment of LOs	Resources
3. Monitor and understand the short-term effects of musculo-skeletal exercise 4. Understand the long-term benefits of musculo-skeletal exercise 5. Know the musculo-skeletal exercise recommendations for young people and where in the community they can perform such exercise	certain strength and flexibility exercises are not recommended (e.g., straight leg sit-ups, standing toe touches, windmills, extreme or rapid arching of the back, bouncing in stretches)		
	Observe and evaluate the exercise technique of others	1	Digital camera, video
	Identify the location and names of the muscles involved (e.g., with curl-ups, straight abdominal muscles are working in the tummy) and monitor and explain the short-term effects of regular strength and flexibility exercises (e.g., improvements in muscular strength and endurance, muscle tone and posture; increases in flexibility, such as the range of movement around joints; gains in ease of performing everyday actions such as lifting, lowering, carrying, reaching, bending, twisting and turning)	2, 3	Differentiated circuit cards, worksheets or record cards, mats, light resistance equipment, benches, rulers, measuring tapes, music machine, music tapes or CDs
	Explain the long-term benefits of performing regular strength and flexibility exercises (e.g., reduced risk of back pain and osteoporosis; improved management of arthritis; increased energy use by toned muscles contributes towards maintenance of a healthy body weight; enhanced fitness for performance such as being able to kick or throw a ball farther and with more power)	4	Posters, charts, CD-ROMs, videos
	Become aware of the musculo-skeletal exercise recommendations for young people (at least twice a week) and discuss where they can perform activities that help to enhance and maintain muscular strength and flexibility and bone health (e.g., PE lessons, at home, exercise classes, sports clubs, gym)	5	Exercise videos, advertisements about local classes

Example Focused Unit: Delivering HRE at Key Stage 4

Aerobics	National curriculum links	
YEAR 10 **Objectives** This unit should enable pupils to do the following: • Perform a range of safe and effective aerobics steps and actions with good technique (including cardiovascular and musculo-skeletal exercise)	**ENGLAND** **Knowledge and understanding of fitness and health** Pupils should be taught how preparation, training and fitness relate to and affect performance; how to design and carry out activity and training programmes that have specific purposes; how exercise and activity will improve personal, social	**WALES** **Exercise activities** Pupils should be taught to refine their techniques and evaluate their performance in at least one activity and to set targets, monitor and evaluate their progress against goals. Pupils should be given opportunities to develop personal and social skills through adopting different roles in a selected activity.

Aerobics	National curriculum links	
• Plan, perform and evaluate the components of an aerobics class • Understand and apply the principles associated with designing, carrying out, monitoring and developing a safe and effective aerobics workout • Have access to physical activity personnel, facilities or services within the local community	and mental health and well-being; and how to monitor and develop their training, exercise and activity programmes in and out of school. **PSHE** Pupils should be taught to be aware of and assess their personal qualities, skills, achievements and potential so that they can set personal goals; to think about the alternatives and long- and short-term consequences when making decisions about personal health; to understand the link between eating patterns and self-image, including eating disorders; to seek professional advice confidently and find information about health; and to recognise and follow health and safety requirements and develop the skills to cope with emergency situations that require basic first aid procedures, including resuscitation techniques.	**Health-related exercise** Pupils should be taught to plan, perform, monitor and evaluate a safe and effective health-related exercise programme that meets their personal needs and preferences over an extended period and to know, understand and be able to demonstrate a practical understanding of the key principles of exercise programming and training, including progression, overload, specificity, balance/moderation/variety, maintenance and reversibility. They should be given opportunities to explore how to overcome constraints to being active, gain access to activity opportunities both in school and in the local community, and appreciate the exercise effects, health benefits and safety issues associated with their selected activities.

Learning outcomes (LOs)	Learning activities	Assessment of LOs	Resources
Pupils should be able to do the following: 1. Perform with good technique a variety of aerobics steps and actions (including cardiovascular, flexibility and strength exercises) 2. Plan and perform a linked series of exercises for each component of an aerobics class 3. Evaluate exercises within an aerobics class in terms of their safety, appropriateness and effectiveness	This unit should provide opportunities for pupils to do the following:		
	Identify and understand the purpose of the different components of an aerobics class (warm-up, cardiovascular section, muscular strength and endurance section, cool-down) and perform a series of exercises with good technique for each component	1	Music machine, tapes or CDs, mats, posters
	Explain safety issues associated with aerobics (e.g., wearing supportive footwear, holding stretches still, avoiding prolonged high-impact exercises, offering alternatives for different abilities)	3	Posters, task cards video, digital camera
	Select and perform appropriate levels of exercises (e.g., from easy, moderate, demanding versions)	3	Music machine, tapes or CDs, mats
	Work with others to plan and perform a series of exercises for each component of an aerobics class (warm-up, cardiovascular section, muscular strength and endurance section, cool-down) and develop personal and social skills through leading part of an aerobics session	2	Music machine, tapes or CDs, mats, task cards

(continued)

Learning outcomes (LOs)	Learning activities	Assessment of LOs	Resources
4. Demonstrate understanding of the principles of exercise programming 5. Have access to community personnel, facilities or services	Explain the principles of exercise programming in developing an aerobics workout (overload, progression, specificity, reversibility)	4	Posters, prompt sheets, task cards
	Set targets, monitor and evaluate progress against goals (e.g., general toning, improved cardiovascular fitness, increased flexibility, weight management)	4	Sportstesters, monitoring equipment, record cards
	Know where to participate in aerobics within the community or at home (e.g., personal workout, videos) and whom to contact for more information	5	Notices, brochures, leaflets, directory, videos, Internet

Example Unit: Delivering HRE Through Athletics at Key Stage 4

Athletics

National curriculum links

YEAR 10

Objectives

This unit should enable pupils to do the following:

- Refine their techniques, strategies and tactics and evaluate their performance in selected running, jumping and throwing events
- Plan, perform, monitor and evaluate effective personal training programmes for their selected events, showing understanding of the principles involved
- Improve performance in selected events
- Adopt different roles for selected events
- Apply safe exercise principles and procedures and evaluate their own and others' warm-ups and cool-downs

ENGLAND

Athletics programme of study

Pupils should be taught to take part in specific athletic events and use advanced techniques and skills with precision, speed, power or stamina and technical proficiency.

Knowledge and understanding of fitness and health

Pupils should be taught how preparation, training and fitness relate to and affect performance; how to design and carry out activity and training programmes that have specific purposes; how exercise and activity improves personal, social and mental health and well-being; and how to monitor and develop their training, exercise and activity programmes in and out of school.

WALES

Sport programme of study

Pupils should be taught to refine their techniques, strategies and tactics as appropriate and evaluate their performance; to develop personal and social skills through adopting different roles in a selected activity; and to understand the role of rules in competition. Pupils should be given opportunities to prepare for taking part in a competitive sports event through training, practice, setting targets and helping to plan the organisation of the sports event.

Health-related exercise

Pupils should be taught to know, understand and demonstrate a practical understanding of the key principles of exercise programming and training, including progression, overload, specificity, balance/moderation/variety, maintenance and reversibility. They should be given opportunities to appreciate the exercise effects, health benefits and safety issues associated with their selected activities.

Learning outcomes (LOs)	Learning activities	Assessment of LOs	Resources
Pupils should be able to do the following: 1. Demonstrate advanced techniques and improved performance in selected running, jumping and throwing events 2. Plan, perform, monitor and evaluate effective personal training programmes for their selected events 3. Demonstrate understanding of the principles of overload, progression, specificity and reversibility within their personal training programmes 4. Adopt different roles (e.g., coach, official) for selected events 5. Apply safe exercise principles and procedures and evaluate their own and others' warm-ups and cool-downs	This unit should provide opportunities for pupils to do the following:		
	Progress from simpler to more advanced techniques, skills and tactics (e.g., developing an approach run or turn for a jumping or throwing event), practise these in competition with themselves and others (as appropriate), and record their progress (e.g., measuring times or distances, noting technical improvements)	1	Equipment for specific events involved (e.g., throwing implements) and for practice (e.g., quoits, hoops, basketballs, canes)
	Take on the role of a coach by being responsible for motivating, observing, evaluating and monitoring improvement in a partner's technique and performance and act as an official for a specific event, demonstrating knowledge of the rules and regulations involved	4	Task cards, prompt sheets, digital camera, video, measuring tapes, watches
	Understand how running, jumping and throwing actions can be improved (e.g., made more powerful) by developing strength and flexibility in particular muscle groups and identify these for selected events (e.g., for discus throw: quadriceps, obliques, pectorals)	3	Muscle and skeleton posters, visual aids, CD-ROMs
	Identify the energy systems predominantly used (i.e., aerobic or anaerobic) in selected events	3	Posters, CD-ROMs
	Understand how training programmes can be progressed by gradually increasing frequency and duration of sessions and the intensity of the exercises (i.e., applying overload and progression), discuss specificity by comparing training programmes for contrasting events, and discuss reversibility by considering the effects of returning to a training programme after a break (e.g., because of illness)	3	Task cards, prompt sheets, personal record cards
	Evaluate the safety, effectiveness and relevance of their own and others' warm-ups and cool-downs	5	Task cards, prompt sheets
	Plan, perform, monitor and evaluate personal training programmes for specific running, jumping and throwing events, including safe and effective warm-ups, cool-downs, and exercises to develop technique, strength, flexibility and aerobic or anaerobic fitness	2	Personal record cards, task cards, prompt sheets

Example Focused Unit: Delivering HRE at Key Stage 4

Weight-training	National curriculum links	
YEAR 11 **Objectives** This unit should enable pupils to do the following: • Perform a range of weight-training exercises with good technique and understand safety issues associated with using weights • Understand the short-term effects and long-term benefits of weight-training and factors affecting participation • Design, carry out, monitor and develop a personal weight-training programme, demonstrating practical understanding of the principles of training • Take responsibility for their own safe, effective and relevant preparation for and recovery from weight-training	**ENGLAND** **Knowledge and understanding of fitness and health** Pupils should be taught how preparation, training and fitness relate to and affect performance; how to design and carry out activity and training programmes that have specific purposes; how exercise and activity will improve personal, social and mental health and well-being; and how to monitor and develop their own training, exercise and activity programmes in and out of school. **PSHE** Pupils should be taught to be aware of and assess their personal qualities, skills, achievements and potential so that they can set personal goals; to think about the alternatives and long- and short-term consequences when making decisions about personal health; to understand the link between eating patterns and self-image, including eating disorders; to seek professional advice confidently and find information about health; and to recognise and follow health and safety requirements and develop the skills to cope with emergency situations that require basic first aid procedures, including resuscitation techniques.	**WALES** **Exercise activities** Pupils should be taught to refine their techniques and evaluate their performance in at least one activity and set targets, monitor and evaluate their progress against goals. Pupils should be given opportunities to develop personal and social skills through adopting different roles in a selected activity. **Health-related exercise** Pupils should be taught to plan, perform, monitor and evaluate a safe and effective health-related exercise programme that meets their personal needs and preferences over an extended period and to know, understand and be able to demonstrate a practical understanding of the key principles of exercise programming and training. They should be given opportunities to explore how to overcome constraints to being active and to gain access to activity opportunities both in school and in the local community; to appreciate the exercise effects, health benefits and safety issues associated with their selected activities; and to appreciate the risks associated with a sedentary lifestyle and with excessive forms and amounts of exercise.

Learning outcomes (LOs)	Learning activities	Assessment of LOs	Resources
Pupils should be able to do the following: 1. Perform with good technique a range of weight-training exercises, showing understanding of safety issues and of the muscle groups involved 2. Plan, perform and monitor a personal	This unit should provide opportunities for pupils to do the following: Explain safety issues associated with weight-training (e.g., minimise stress on the back, select appropriate levels of exercises, work at your own pace, avoid competition with others, control the lifting and lowering of weights, alternate muscle groups, check the position of pins)	1	Posters, charts, prompt sheets, task cards
	Perform a range of weight-training exercises with safe and effective technique and identify	1	Weights (free or fixed), dumb-bells,

Learning outcomes (LOs)	Learning activities	Assessment of LOs	Resources
weight-training programme over a period of four to six weeks, showing understanding of the principles of training 3. Understand the short-term effects and long-term health benefits of weight-training 4. Understand factors affecting participation and know where they can participate in weight-training in the community	the major muscle groups that are working in each exercise		elastics, tubing, circuit cards, muscle and skeleton posters, CD-ROMs
	Observe, evaluate and correct the exercise technique of others	1	Prompt sheets, task cards, video, digital camera
	Demonstrate practical understanding of the principles of training (overload, progression, specificity, reversibility), such as explaining ways overload can be applied (e.g., more repetitions, more sets, increased resistance, decreased rest before working same muscle group again)	2	
	Plan, perform and evaluate a personal weight-training programme that includes a relevant warm-up and cool-down	2	Record cards, personal schedules
	Set targets and evaluate progress against goals (e.g., general toning, weight management) by means of appropriate methods of monitoring their personal weight-training programme (e.g., timed or paced curl-ups; exercise diaries recording sets, repetitions and resistance; written comments about how the exercise feels)	2	Monitoring equipment, record cards, diaries
	Explain the benefits of weight-training (e.g., improves muscle tone, assists weight management, reduces risk of back pain and osteoporosis; can be done alone; not weather dependent) and the constraints (e.g., cost, time, risk of injury if safety issues are ignored, myths about negative effects of weight-training)	3,4	Posters, charts, CD-ROMs, task cards
	Find out and discuss where they can take part in weight-training (e.g., school, home, youth club, leisure centre, fitness club)	4	Notices, brochures, leaflets, directory Internet

Example Focused Unit: Delivering HRE at Key Stage 4

Personal exercise programme	National curriculum links	
YEAR 11	**ENGLAND**	**WALES**
Objectives This unit should enable pupils to do the following: • Plan, perform, monitor and evaluate a safe and effective health-related exercise programme that meets their personal needs and preferences over an extended period	**Knowledge and understanding of fitness and health** Pupils should be taught how preparation, training and fitness relate to and affect performance; how to design and carry out activity and training programmes that have specific purposes; how exercise and activity will improve personal, social	**Exercise activities** Pupils should be taught to refine their techniques and evaluate their performance in at least one activity and to set targets, monitor and evaluate their progress against goals. Pupils should be given opportunities to develop personal and social skills *(continued)*

Personal exercise programme	**National curriculum links**	
YEAR 11	**ENGLAND**	**WALES**
• Demonstrate a practical understanding of the principles of exercise programming • Consider constraints to being active and how to overcome them and appreciate the risks associated with a sedentary lifestyle and with excessive amounts of exercise Sections of this unit are delivered within the PSHE-PSE programme.	and mental health and well-being; and how to monitor and develop their training, exercise and activity programmes in and out of school. **PSHE** Pupils should be taught to be aware of and assess their personal qualities, skills, achievements and potential so that they can set personal goals; to think about the alternatives and long- and short-term consequences when making decisions about personal health; to understand the link between eating patterns and self-image, including eating disorders; to seek professional advice confidently and find information about health; and to recognise and follow health and safety requirements.	through adopting different roles in a selected activity. **Health-related exercise** Pupils should be taught to plan, perform, monitor and evaluate a safe and effective health-related exercise programme that meets their personal needs and preferences over an extended period and to know, understand and be able to demonstrate a practical understanding of the key principles of exercise programming. They should be given opportunities to explore how to overcome constraints to being active and to gain access to activity opportunities both in school and in the local community and to appreciate the risks associated with a sedentary lifestyle and with excessive forms and amounts of exercise.

Learning outcomes (LOs)	**Learning activities**	**Assessment of LOs**	**Resources**
Pupils should be able to do the following: 1. Plan an exercise programme that meets their personal needs and preferences 2. Perform, monitor and evaluate a personal exercise programme over a period of time 3. Demonstrate practical understanding of the principles of exercise programming 4. Propose ways of overcoming constraints to being active and understand the risks involved in	This unit should provide opportunities for pupils to do the following: Identify within a personal profile their needs and preferences and assess their qualities, skills, achievements and potential so that they can set personal goals to help them follow activity recommendations and develop a commitment to an active lifestyle (PSHE)	1	Personal profiles, posters, charts, CD-ROM
	Evaluate a range of activities in terms of appeal, accessibility (e.g., cost, travel, reliance on others) and effectiveness in developing fitness components (PSHE)	1	Personal profiles, posters, charts, CD-ROM
	Design and carry out a personal exercise programme from a selection of accessible activities in and out of school (e.g., walking, jogging, cycling, dancing, sport, aqua exercise, skipping, circuits), including safe, effective warm-up and cool-down routines (PE)	2	Equipment appropriate to the activities
	Explain how their personal exercise programme progresses over a period of weeks and how they are monitoring their progress (e.g., activity diary, practical monitoring procedures such as fitness tests) (PE)	2, 3	Activity diaries, monitoring equipment

Learning outcomes (LOs)	Learning activities	Assessment of LOs	Resources
sedentary living and in extreme health behaviours	Demonstrate understanding of the principles of exercise programming including the desirability of balance and variety in the programme and the need for moderation and consideration of how to maintain involvement (PE)	3	Prompt sheets, task cards, posters, charts, personal profiles
	Discuss constraints to being active (e.g., cost, time, travel) and propose ways of overcoming them (e.g., exercising at home, walking or cycling to school) (PSHE)	4	Prompt sheets, task cards, posters, charts, personal profiles
	Explain the risks associated with a sedentary lifestyle (e.g., increased risk of heart disease, obesity, osteoporosis, back pain, stress) and with extreme forms of dieting and exercising (e.g., developing eating disorders) (PSHE)	4	Prompt sheets, task cards, posters, charts, personal profiles

Appendix A

Health-Related Exercise Resources

American Master Teacher Program (1994). *Teaching children fitness.* (30-minute video). Champaign, IL: Human Kinetics.

Armstrong, N. (1991). Health-related physical activity. In N. Armstrong and A. Sparkes (Eds.), *Issues in physical education.* (pp. 139–154). London: Cassell Educational Ltd.

Armstrong, N., and Welsman, J. (1997). *Young people and physical activity.* Oxford University Press.

Awdurdod Cymwysterau Cwricwlwm Ac Asesu Cymru (ACCAC) (1997). *Health-related exercise posters.* (Primary set and Secondary set). Aberystwyth: Francis Balsom Associates, Number 4 The Science Park, Aberystwyth, Ceredigion SY23 3AH. Telephone: 01970-611996. Fax: 01970-625796.

Awdurdod Cymwysterau Cwricwlwm Ac Asesu Cymru (ACCAC) (2000). *Health-related exercise at key stage 3—pupil task cards and teacher's handbook.* Aberystwyth: Francis Balsom Associates, Number 4 The Science Park, Aberystwyth, Ceredigion SY23 3AH. Telephone: 01970-611996. Fax: 01970-625796.

Biddle, S. (1991). Promoting health-related physical activity in schools. In N. Armstrong and A. Sparkes (Eds.), *Issues in physical education.* (pp. 155–169). London: Cassell Educational Ltd.

Biddle, S., Sallis, J., and Cavill, N. (Eds.) (1998). *Young and active? Young people and health-enhancing physical activity—evidence and implications*. London: Health Education Authority.

Bodycare Products Ltd. (1990). *Set of posters: The skeletal system; the muscular system.* Available from Bodycare Products Ltd., Unit 9A, Princes Drive Industrial Estate, Kenilworth, Warwickshire CV8 2FD.

British Association of Advisers and Lecturers in Physical Education (BAALPE) (1995). *Safe practice in physical education*. Dudley LEA: West Midlands.

British Heart Foundation (1996). *Jump rope for heart health teacher's manual*. London: Author.

British Heart Foundation (1999). *The active school. Resource pack for primary schools*. London: Author.

Cale, L., Clarke, F., Harris, J., McGeorge, S., and McGeorge, C. (1996). *Keep the beat.* London: British Heart Foundation.

Donovan, G., McNamara, J., and Gianoli, P. (1989). *Exercise stop danger.* Hampshire: Fitness Leader Network, PO Box 70, Fareham, Hampshire PO14 4 HT.

Elbourn, J. (1998). *Fit for TOPs*—an addition to the Youth Sport Trust TOPs programme developed by YMCA Fitness Industry Training and supported by the English Sports Council. Loughborough: Youth Sport Trust.

Elbourn, J. (1998). *Planning a personal exercise programme.* London: YMCA Fitness Industry Training.

Elbourn, J., and Brennan, M. (1998). *Assisting a circuit-training instructor.* London: YMCA Fitness Industry Training.

Elbourn, J., and Brennan, M. (1998). *Assisting an exercise to music instructor.* London: YMCA Fitness Industry Training.

Fox, K.R. (1991). Physical education and its contribution to health and well-being. In N. Armstrong and A. Sparkes (Eds.), *Issues in physical education.* (pp.123–138). London: Cassell Educational Ltd.

Harris, J. (1997). A health focus in physical education. In L. Almond (Ed.), *Physical education in schools.* (2nd ed., pp. 104–120). London: Kogan Page.

Harris, J., and Elbourn, J. (1990). *Action for heart health. A practical health related exercise programme for physical education.* Loughborough University, Leicestershire: Exercise and Health Group.

Harris, J., and Elbourn, J. (1991). *Further activity ideas for heart health.* Loughborough University, Leicestershire: Exercise and Health Group.

Harris, J., and Elbourn, J. (1992). *Warming up and cooling down. Practical ideas for implementing the physical education national curriculum.* Loughborough University, Leicestershire: Exercise and Health Group. Available from YMCA Fitness Industry Training.

Harris, J., and Elbourn, J. (1997). *Teaching health-related exercise at key stages 1 and 2.* Champaign, IL: Human Kinetics.

Harris, J., and Elbourn, J. (2001). *Teaching health-related exercise at key stages 3 and 4.* Champaign, IL: Human Kinetics.

Health Education Authority (1997). *Young people and physical activity. A literature review.* London: Author.

Health Education Authority (1997). *Young people and physical activity. Promoting better practice.* London: Author.

Health Education Authority (1998). *Young and active? Policy framework for young people and health-enhancing physical activity*. London: Author.

Health Education Authority (1998). *Young and active presentation pack.* London: Author. ISBN: 0 7521 1292 9. Free from Marstons Book Services; tel: 01235 465 565.

Hopper, C., Fisher, B., and Munoz, K.D. (1997). *Health-related fitness for Grades 1 and 2/3 and 4/5 and 6.* (3 texts). Champaign, IL: Human Kinetics.

Kalbfleisch, S. (1987). *Skip to it. The new skipping book.* London: A and C Black.

McGeorge, S. (1993). *The exercise challenge.* Loughborough University, Leicestershire: Exercise and Health Group.

Mulvihull, C., Rivers, K., and Aggleton, P. (2000). *Physical activity 'at our time'. Qualitative research among young people aged 5 to 15 years and parents.* London: Health Education Authority.

Pate, R.R., and Hohn, R.C. (Eds.) (1994). *Health and fitness through physical education.* Champaign, IL: Human Kinetics.

Puma (1997). *Pro-active. A student resource for physical education at key stage 4.* Northampton: Educational Project Resources Ltd.

Ratliffe, T., and Ratliffe, L.M. (1994). *Teaching children fitness. Becoming a master teacher.* Champaign, IL: Human Kinetics.

Royal Navy (1996). *Royal Marines Commando action fitness health related activity.* Available from The Royal Navy Education Service, PO Box 934, Poole, Dorset BH17 7BR.

Sleap, M. (1994). Fit for life 2. *Physical activity sessions for children aged 7–13 years.* Hull: University of Hull.

University of Hull (1994). *Fitness challenge.* University of Hull and Children's World.

University of Hull (1994). *Take up the fitness challenge. The fun way to a healthier future.* (Video). University of Hull and Children's World.

YMCA Fitness Industry Training (1994). *Getting it right. The Y's guide to safe and effective exercise.* (40-minute video). London: Author.

Appendix B

Health-Related Exercise Contacts

ADDRESSES

Awdurdod Cymwysterau Cwricwlwm Ac Asesu Cymru (ACCAC) (Qualifications, Curriculum and Assessment Authority for Wales)

Castle Buildings
Womanby Street
Cardiff
CF10 9SX
Tel: 01222-375400

Awdurdod Cymwysterau Cwricwlwm Ac Asesu Cymru (ACCAC) Publications (Qualifications, Curriculum and Assessment Authority for Wales Publications)

PO Box 2129
Erdington
Birmingham
B24 ORD
Tel: 07071-223646/7

British Association of Advisers and Lecturers in Physical Education

Nelson House, 6 The Beacon
Exmouth
Devon
EX8 2AG
Tel: 01395-263247

British Association of Sport and Exercise Sciences

114 Cardigan Road
Headingley
Leeds
LS6 3BJ
Tel: 0113-289-1020

British Heart Foundation

14 Fitzhardinge Street
London
W1H 4DH
Tel: 020-7935-0185

British Heart Foundation National Centre for Physical Activity and Health

Department of Physical Education, Sports Science and Recreation Management
Loughborough University
Leics
LE11 3TU
Tel: 01509-223259

Department for Education and Employment Publications

PO Box 5050
Annesley
Nottingham
NG15 ODJ
Tel: 0845-6022260

Health Development Agency (formerly the Health Education Authority)

Trevelyan House
30 Great Peter Street
London
SW1P 2HW
Tel: 020-7222-5300

Health Promotion Division of the National Assembly for Wales

Ffynnon-Las
Ty Glas Avenue
Llanishen
Cardiff
CF14 5EZ
Tel: 01222-752222

Institute of Youth Sport

Rutland Building
Loughborough University
Leics
LE11 3TU
01509-223263

Jump Rope for Heart

National Events Department
British Heart Foundation
14 Fitzhardinge Street
London
W1H 4DH
Tel: 0171-935-0185

National Coaching Foundation

4 College Close
Beckett Park
Leeds
LSU 3QH
Tel: 0113-274-4802

Physical Education Association of the United Kingdom

Ling House, Building 25
London Road
Reading
RG1 5AQ
Tel: 0118-931-6240

Qualifications and Curriculum Authority

29 Bolton Street
London
W1Y 7PD
Tel: 0171-509-5555

Sport England

16 Upper Woburn Place
London
WC1H OQP
Tel: 020-7273-1500

Sports Council for Wales

Sophia Gardens
Cardiff
CF11 9SW
Tel: 01222-300500

YMCA Fitness Industry Training

112 Great Russell Street
London
WC1B 3NQ
Tel: 0171-343-1850

Youth Sport Trust

Rutland Building
Loughborough University
Leics
LE11 3TU
Tel: 01509-228290/1/2

WEB SITES

Wired for Health

www.wiredforhealth.gov.uk

Physical activity Web site for teenagers

www.NRgize.co.uk